7 Days of Being Kinder to Yourself

Marie Glaeser

7 Days of Being Kinder to Yourself

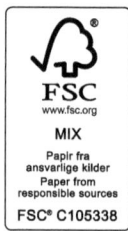

Forlag: BoD – Books on Demand, København, Danmark

Tryk: BoD – Books on Demand, Norderstedt, Tyskland

ISBN: 9788743014072

To Trish, who I wish could have read this book.

Table of Contents

Introduction

we don't
expect a plant to grow
when we don't
give it water,
sunshine
soil
or food

so why do we
expect to grow
when we don't
care
for ourselves?

I'm so happy you are here, reading this book.

I wrote it for those of you who want to spend a week taking good care of yourself – to see what happens when you do.

Those who want to build new habits in the way you eat, think and get up in the morning – to see what happens when you do. Those of you who are feeling low, stressed, overwhelmed or get up with a knot in your stomach each morning. Those who have no idea how to make room for all the *good for you* things you hear about. Those of you whose internal voice is your worst critic, a never-ending stream of unkind thoughts.

I wrote it for you if you want to re-discover the joy of good food, good sleep, friendships, kindness, movement, the outdoors and all the other pleasures the world has to offer.

This little book will accompany you for 21 meals and seven days. Each morning it will greet you with words of encouragement and a challenge for the day. It will also ask you to write down some things you are grateful for each morning. There will be daily recipes for breakfast, lunch and dinner, as well as a snack inspiration if you need it. Each evening this book provides a space for you to reflect on the day, how you found the challenge and to write down one (or a few) things you learned that day.

At the back of this book, you will find the entire week's meal plan, as well as a shopping list of what you will need. I would recommend you make sure you have everything on this list before you start working through the book.

This book is for people with all sorts of different amounts of time, money, physical challenges and energy, dietary patterns and access to shops and products – that means I have tried to provide a few options for each recipe. I hope this means that getting what you need to follow through with this week's plan is manageable, but if it isn't – then take it as your first challenge to think of some alternatives that you could buy/make/eat this week.

I have provided 19 different recipes so that you have several inspirations for new meals to include in your routine. This doesn't mean you have to make 19 different recipes this week! If you particularly like one recipe you can just make it on a few days, whilst skipping those that don't interest you.

A note on feelings
Recognising the role of emotions

I am writing this book to help you spend a week engaging in practices that improve your wellbeing. I am not writing this book to stop you from feeling sad, angry, scared or stressed.

Before you close this book and say 'That's not what I am looking for, I want to stop feeling those things.' keep reading for a little longer to understand why this book isn't written to help you stop feeling those things.

Feelings and emotions have a purpose [1]. Read that again. Feelings and emotions have a purpose. Always.

When something bad happens to us, such as losing a family member, we grieve. Grieving allows us to say goodbye to that person and to seek support from loved ones around us in a time where we need more social connection. When we are in a dangerous situation, such as getting into a car with a drunk driver, we may feel scared. Fear allows to consider the consequences of a situation and to help keep us safe by changing the situation.

The problem with depression, stress and anxiety is that we don't always know *why* we are feeling that way. When there is no concrete cause we conclude that we must be feeling that way because something is wrong with us, our world or our life.

I would argue that's not true. But your feelings are not wrong either. Because feelings and emotions have a purpose.

If a child was sad, what would your natural instinct be? It is likely that you would comfort her, say nice things to her, give her cuddles, distract her with a fun activity.

If a child was scared, what would your natural instinct be? It is likely that you would try and find out what exactly he is scared of, then you would encourage him, help him solve the problem or offer him support in doing what he is scared of.

The needs that are expressed by these emotions may be social connection, support, comfort, encouragement or many other things. These emotions have a purpose.

When you are sad or scared, what is your natural instinct? It is likely that you tell yourself off, that you tell yourself something is wrong with you for feeling this way, that you can never solve the problem, that there is no point trying to change anything or that nobody around you will understand or help. Or you might try and push the emotion away, force it to be silent.

There are three things that are important to keep in mind.

1. Your emotions have a purpose. And I'm aware I am repeating myself here, but I need this to sink in. Throughout the coming week practice noticing your emotions and trying to understand the need behind them. Then think about how you could meet that need. It is okay to feel sad or stressed or scared or angry. *Try to treat yourself as you would treat a child or a friend experiencing your emotions.*

2. You may also have other feelings. These may include feeling worthless, like a failure, ashamed, inadequate, useless and so on. These feelings are often related to the way we think and on day 2 of this journal we will look at how this affects you in more detail. For now, I would just like to point out the difference between an emotion having a purpose (such as grief or sadness) and an emotion meaning something is a fact. So, for example, feeling like a failure does not mean you *are* a failure. Feeling alone does not mean you *are* alone. Feeling scared does not mean there *is* definitely danger. Feeling incompetent does not mean you can't do something. *Throughout this week practice recognising your feelings as feelings and noticing when you are interpreting them as facts.*

3. The more we try to push away an emotion the more we feel it [2]. It's like trying to hold a ball filled with air under water – have you ever tried that? On the other hand, the more we try to hold on to an emotion the more likely it is to dissipate. Trying to hold on to a feeling is like trying to hold on to smoke with your hands. *Throughout this week practice noticing your emotions and leaving them as they are.* Notice where you feel them in your body, notice how they shift and change, notice what happens when you turn your attention from the emotion back onto the activity you are currently doing.

A note on circumstance

Recognising the role of live events.

Whilst it is true that we don't always know why we feel the way we feel when we are anxious or depressed [3], [4], sometimes we know exactly why.

Your situation right now might be extremely difficult and could be the cause of how you are feeling. Actually about 80% of people struggling with depression have faced one or more difficult life events that could have triggered their depression [5].

Common causes are job insecurity, job stress, relationship difficulties, divorce, loss, financial problems, problems with accommodation, social isolation, ill health and being a carer for someone who is ill [4], [5]. Other factors that can play a role include having too much or too little responsibility at work, your commute, past experiences, travel, moving house, getting married, changing work and much more [4], [5].

These are things that you might be going through right now, or things that happened to you in the distant or recent past [5]. Sometimes we cope incredibly well during a difficult situation, only to feel completely unable to face the day weeks after the situation has already past.

This book focuses on things you can *do* right now to take care of yourself in or after difficult situations. It introduces thought experiments that can help you think differently about these situations or to shift your focus away from thinking about them.

It does these things not because the way you think or spend your days necessarily *caused* your feelings. It isn't trying to resolve the situation you are experiencing or experienced, it isn't trying to say that what you have gone through was 'not so bad'.

Not at all.

The reason this book focuses on those things is that those are the things you *can change*. You may not be able to change your current situation right now, you definitely can't change what happened in the past and you can't predict the future. But you can make damn sure to take the best possible care of yourself *right now*. You can make sure you are in the best possible place to work through whatever it is you are going through right now.

Think of it this way – if you were planning a cross country road trip from North Africa all the way down to South Africa – what would you do with your car before you start the journey? I'm guessing you would fuel up, check the oil, change the tyres and organise a spare set, check the engine is in the best possible condition and so on. We know that a car needs to be in good condition to get through a long, difficult journey safely.

The problem is that we often forget that we, and our bodies, also need to be in good condition to get through long, difficult journeys.

Take a moment to write down some of the life circumstances that you feel are affecting you at the moment:

Recognise what you are dealing with. Now turn the pages to begin focusing on how to care for yourself on this journey.

Some practical things

- Always make sure that any fruits and vegetables you use have been well washed.
- Having said that, I recommend not peeling your vegetables because the peel contains fibre and nutrients.
- Make sure you don't mix up raw meats or animal products with foods that you will be eating uncooked.
- You usually know your pan is hot enough when the oil fizzes if you press a wooden spoon against it.
- The recipes in this book might be higher in fibre than you are used to. This can lead to bloating, gassiness or digestive discomfort in the beginning, but should get better with time. If you have any concerns always speak to your doctor or health care professional.
- When you eat more fibre, it is really important that you also drink enough water to make sure you don't get constipated – this means drinking at least 8 glasses of water a day!
- To make finding alternatives easier where the recipes I provide don't meet your current needs each recipe contains some foods which fall into certain categories. At the back of this book you can find a list of alternatives for each of the categories.
- The portion sizes in this book result in you eating around 2000kcal per day.
- This may not be enough for you, particularly if you are a man, very active or large, growing or pregnant. On the other hand, it may be too much for you. *Please listen to your body as you work through this book and increase or decrease portion sizes as needed.*

3 Key Concepts

Introducing the science this book is based on

You may be wondering why you should care about food if you are feeling low, anxious or stressed. Surely food is for physical wellbeing and a therapist is for your mental wellbeing?

Let's carry out a small thought experiment to consider how food might affect you subjectively. Afterwards I will introduce you to some of the science behind the links between food and mood. Consider the questions below:

- How do you feel when you have not eaten anything all day?
- How do you feel when you have grazed on snacks and junk food all day?
- How do you feel when you have drunk 6 cups of coffee in a day?
- How do you feel when you have spent the evening snacking on foods right up until the moment you go to bed?
- How do you feel when you skip breakfast?
- How do you feel if you had your lunch at your desk whilst working?
- How do you feel when you have had a healthy breakfast?
- How do you feel after a delicious home-cooked meal surrounded by family or friends?
- How do you feel when you have had time for your lunch and ate it outside in the sun?
- How do you feel when you cook yourself a dinner from scratch?

Of course, I don't know you. But my own experience and the experience of many people I have worked with tells me that the first six options will likely make you feel all sorts of unhelpful physical and mental effects. You might feel lethargic, tired, jumpy, on edge, guilty, anxious, bloated, uncomfortable and so on. The final four options are likely to leave you feeling energised, happy, virtuous, loved and taken care of.

Now – that's not the case all the time. But in general, certain ways of eating leave you with a feeling of well-being, whilst others contribute to you feeling the opposite. Often, we get into a vicious cycle because feeling low or stressed is likely to make us skip meals, eat convenience foods, comfort eat or graze, drink too much caffeine or eat on the go. This book will hopefully help you break some of those habits even if you are not feeling well.

In addition, the recipes focus on supporting you in three key areas, which have been linked with mental health. In this section I will tell you about the links between blood sugar, inflammation, the gut and your mental wellbeing.

You absolutely don't need to read or understand them to benefit from the book. On the other hand – it may help you understand the reasons behind some of the things I suggest, which may make it easier for you to continue making changes after the end of the 7 days.

Blood Sugar

Blood sugar balance is a term that is becoming well-known. When we eat, foods are broken down into smaller molecules by our digestive system, which are then absorbed into our blood stream. One of these molecules is glucose, which comes particularly from carbohydrates. The amount of glucose in the blood stream is known as your blood sugar.

Blood sugar is important as it is one of our primary sources of energy [1] – and so our bodies try to keep our blood sugar levels within a very tightly regulated range [2]. Diabetes is a condition that occurs when the body loses its ability to keep blood sugar within this range[3].

Insulin resistance plays a key role in the development of type 2 Diabetes (which, unlike type 1 Diabetes, is a result of lifestyle and environment) [4]. Insulin is the hormone that the body releases to tell your cells to take up blood sugar, lowering blood sugar levels and providing your cells with energy to function [2]. A variety of factors can lead to cells no longer responding to insulin, which means they no longer open up for the blood sugar [2]. This results in elevated sugar levels in the blood stream, whilst the cells lack energy to function [5]. This is known as insulin resistance [2].

Interestingly, diabetes almost doubles your chance of experiencing depression [3]. Additionally, treating depression with serotonin reuptake inhibitor antidepressants leads to an improvement in blood sugar regulation as well as an improvement in symptoms of depression [3]. Furthermore, stress inhibits insulin [5]. That means when you are stressed it is more difficult for your body to regulate blood sugar and its' levels are more likely to spike [5]. All this points towards some sort of relationship between blood sugar regulation and mood.

I'm going to tell you about three possible explanations of this relationship:

1. *The first and simpler reason* is that the physical symptoms of low and high blood sugar mimic the physical symptoms of low mood, stress and anxiety. Go through the lists below and underline any physical feelings you recognise from when you felt low, stressed or anxious:

High blood sugar:
- frequent need to pee
- lack of energy
- stomach pain
- weight gain
- nausea
- vomiting (when it's really bad)
- getting ill frequently [6]

Low blood sugar:
- sweating
- tingling limbs
- shaking
- dizziness
- lack of energy
- fatigue
- racing heart
- difficulty concentrating and solving problems
- sleepiness
- increased irritability
- anxiety
- moodiness
- feeling tearful
- paleness [2], [5], [7].

Interesting right?

Now I'm not saying that your depression or anxiety are purely a result of this, but I absolutely think it can feed into a vicious cycle. Particularly when you think about how low mood and anxiety can affect your eating – skipping meals, reaching for quick convenience foods that might trigger a blood sugar spike (more about this later in the book) – leading to high or low blood sugar and the resulting physical feelings will only make you feel lower or more anxious.

For example – you may need to give a presentation at work which you are nervous about. As a result of this nervousity you skip breakfast and simply grab a coffee before work. The caffeine from the coffee will briefly lead to a rise in blood sugar, followed by a quick drop because of the lack of other foods. By the time you come to your presentation your blood sugar is likely to be low, so you might be shaking, nauseous and irritable. Because you don't know this is due to your blood sugar you will think it is because you are so nervous – and you may think you are so nervous because you are not equipped to give the presentation. This will make you more nervous, and the resulting anxiety will probably exacerbate your shaking and nausea and so on.

2. *The second reason* is that low blood sugar can trigger the release of catecholamines, which are our stress hormones [2]. Their function is to enhance the release of stored glucose from liver and muscle cells – which is important as very low blood sugar can be dangerous and lead to death [2]. However, an increase in stress hormones is also likely to increase your perceived stress levels.

Another stress hormone, cortisol, is likely to be increased during stressful periods. This hormone not only enhances the effect of catecholamines, but it also inhibits insulin and increases glucose levels in the body by enhancing the conversion of proteins into stored glucose (known as glucagon) [2]. Therefore, during periods in which you are stressed you may be more likely to experience elevated blood sugar levels – and this important because of the third link between blood sugar and mental wellbeing, which I describe next.

3. *The third, and slightly more complex reason* is that elevated blood sugar leads to increased levels of inflammation. An increase in blood glucose following a meal leads to increased expression of a particular pro-inflammatory cytokine (or chemical messenger), which plays an important role in triggering the release of insulin [8]. Whilst this is generally a normal response to eating, it is important to note that the amount of the inflammatory cytokine that is released is directly dependent on the amount of glucose detected in the bloodstream [8]. Therefore, the higher the blood sugar, the higher the level of pro-inflammatory messaging.

High levels of glucose in the brain can also have an inflammatory effect, which can in fact lead to neurological damage [9]. Ironically, this damage leads to a loss of the cells which usually regulate brain glucose – and so the likelihood of increased brain glucose and therefore inflammation is increased [9].

In one study rats on a high sugar diet exhibited rapidly increased inflammation in comparison to rats on a normal or a high fat and sugar diet [10]. The authors concluded that this was a result of sugar induced hyperglycaemia (or high blood sugar) [10]. Research indicates that the combination of high fat, high sugar diets has a particularly bad impact on insulin sensitivity and inflammation [11]–[13].

Inflammation matters because research is increasingly finding a link between stress, low mood, anxiety and increased levels of inflammation. I will talk about what this link might be in the next section so read on.

There may be other explanations of why there is a relationship between blood sugar regulation and your mental health, but these are the three that I come across most often. I should also highlight that research is still unclear on the cause-effect nature of the relationship. It might be that poor blood sugar regulation and increased inflammation cause low mood or anxiety, or low mood and anxiety cause blood sugar dysregulation and inflammation. Or – that the relationship between these factors is multi-directional.

Regardless, the recipes and snack ideas I give you in this book are all aimed at making it easier for your body to regulate blood sugar. Although everyone's reaction to what they eat will be individual, I have used research findings to design recipes that provide your body with energy that is released slowly, over time – preventing the risk of blood sugar spikes and energy dips.

Inflammation

Elevated markers of inflammation have been found time and time again in individuals experiencing depression [14]–[16], stress [17], [18] or anxiety [19]–[21].

Research is not yet clear on whether inflammation causes these mood states, or the mood states cause inflammation, or whether the two affect each other in a bi-directional relationship.

There is however budding research, which indicates that reducing inflammation through reducing the 'inflammatory load' of the diet can have a positive impact on mood states.

One study, conducted only with women, found that the greater the inflammatory load of the diet, the greater the risk of having depression 12 years later [22]. In another large cross-sectional study a significant relationship was found between the inflammatory load of the diet and current symptoms of depression, anxiety and generally reduced wellbeing [23]. I should mention that these studies did not measure physiological markers of inflammation, but simply concluded from the reported diets that there may be an increase in these markers.

A study conducted with rats found that 16 weeks of a high fat diet led to increased levels of inflammatory markers and induced anxiety behaviours [24]. Other studies have found that omega-3 supplementation, which can have anti-inflammatory effects, improves treatment response in depressed individuals with high levels of inflammation at baseline [25], [26].

Inflammation also increases the likelihood of insulin resistance [27], which, as we discussed above, can lead to the physical symptoms of high blood sugar. Furthermore, as you now know; high blood sugar increases inflammation – and so we have a vicious cycle where inflammation increases blood sugar and increased blood sugar increases inflammation.

Inflammation triggers 'sickness' behaviours, which include withdrawing, increased need to sleep and rest and changes in eating behaviours [28], it also results in changes in neurotransmitter (the chemical messengers in our brains) balance, which might affect those neurotransmitters that contribute to happy mood, motivation or calmness (such as serotonin)) [9], [29].

Research shows that diets high in refined sugars and carbohydrates, saturated fats and low in whole, fresh plant foods can be pro-inflammatory [30], [31]. Diets similar to the Mediterranean diet, which are high in whole plant foods such as fresh fruit and vegetables, whole-grains and legumes, as well as unsaturated fats such as olive oil, and a moderate amount of fish and unprocessed meat, can be anti-inflammatory [32].

The recipes you will find in this book incorporate a variety of fresh, whole plant foods, oily fish and unprocessed meat in order to support your body in regulating inflammation.

The Gut

The final factor I would like to tell you about is the gut. More and more research is focusing on identifying how the little bacteria guys living in your gut (I will refer to them as gut bugs from now on) affect mood and anxiety. You have more gut bug cells in your gut than you have human cells, in fact, together your gut bugs weigh between 1 and 2kg, which is basically the same weight as your brain [33]! The more we learn about these little guys, the more we understand that they play a huge role in our well-being, affecting far more than just our digestion.

There is increasing recognition of the gut-brain connection, which not only means that the brain can send messages to the gut, but also that the gut can send messages to the brain [33].

The brain for example may send the gut the message to stop all digestive function when you are in a dangerous situation – this is necessary to help you invest all your energy into fighting off danger or running away [33]. The gut sends a multitude of messages to the brain, including immune signals, neurotransmitters (such as Serotonin, which I mentioned yesterday) and even food cravings [33]!

The gut bugs play a key role in regulating this communication. How they do this is a really good question that we don't have a definite answer to yet. But we do know for example, that exposure to stress changes which bugs thrive in your gut and what kinds of metabolic products they release. This can lead to you being more sensitive to stress and experiencing more anxiety [33], perhaps because the products they release send signals to the brain (via your immune system or your vagus nerve) [33], [34].

Gut bugs also affect the way the brain develops (particularly in babies [35]), and they can upregulate the production of our 'happy neurotransmitter' serotonin in the cells lining our gut [36]–[38]. Research is increasingly indicating that through all these different pathways the health of the gut has a big impact on our mental wellbeing – which might also partly explain why individuals suffering from chronic digestive conditions such as IBS are so much more likely to experience depression or low mood [36]. Finally, gut bugs can increase or decrease inflammation in the body – which as you now know plays a role in mood [39].

The problem with all of this is that we don't yet know what the ideal gut bugs are to have – and in what quantities we need them. In fact, the more we learn the more it seems like there is not one answer to this question – it seems different things are ideal for different people.
The one thing that we do keep noting is that the more different types of bugs we have the better (usually) [38]. Think about it like a garden – if the plants you want to have there are thriving there is much less room for weeds.

Foods that seem to encourage diversity are foods that also help in regulating blood sugar and inflammation – they are colourful, whole foods high in fibre and polyphenols (which give plant foods their rich colours) [38], [40]–[42]. Perhaps unsurprisingly then, diets high in these foods are also associated with a reduced likelihood of depression [40].

The recipes in this book are all designed to provide lots of 'fertiliser' for a diverse range of gut bugs. Across the 7 days you will eat a variety of different fruits, vegetables and whole-grains – providing you with plenty of fibre and phytonutrients.

How to use this book

The remainder of this book is set up like a journal and cookbook. For seven days you will find a morning greeting, recipes for the day and daily cognitive behavioural therapy or mindfulness challenges. Think of it as a 7-day challenge to be kind to yourself.

Choose a week where you will have time (or are able to make time) to follow the routines and recipes set out in this book. I recommend you use the weekend to shop and prepare, so you can start your at home retreat on a Monday (assuming you work Monday-Friday).

During this week make time to answer the questions and challenges set out in the journal by writing your answers down – either in this book or in a separate notebook.

Note: Skip to page 30 the evening before you start the challenge to prepare your breakfast for the first day. You may also want to skip to page 32 in order to prepare your lunch.

Make sure you have bought all the ingredients set out in the shopping list on page 99, before you intend to start the 7-day challenge.

DISCLAIMER: None of the information provided in this book is intended to diagnose, treat or cure any medical or mental health conditions. Always consult your medical practitioner before making any significant changes to your diet, lifestyle or similar. The information in this book is not intended to suggest that you should not seek professional advice or follow your medical professional's recommendations. It is always best to make lifestyle changes under the care of a medically trained practitioner.

"I know that there is nothing better for people than to be
happy and to do good while they live.

That each of them may eat and drink, and find
satisfaction in all their toil
– this is the gift of God."

Ecclesiastes 3, 12-13

Good morning,

I am glad you are here today, and I hope you slept well?

Take a moment to check in with your body – how does it
feel this morning? Is it tired, achy and heavy? Do you
have a knot in your stomach or chest? Or are you feeling
energetic and light?

What do you think your body needs today, to help take
care of it, based on how it is feeling right now?

Your first challenge for this week is to try and do what
you have just written down for your body today. It might
be to take a bath this evening, to go for a walk or a run, to
drink herbal tea instead of your third cup of coffee, to
take a shower or to wear some nice clothes today. It may
also be something completely different, go with your gut
instinct on what your body is asking for – and do it.

Before you head off to make your breakfast, take some
time to write down what you are grateful for today:

*"Gratefulness – a sense of wonder, appreciation and
thankfulness"* [43]

Gratefulness

Things you might be grateful for include your home, your family, your body, your health, your friends, your work – or grander scheme things like the sun, the birds, that there is peace in your country. It does not have to be something specific that has happened recently, it is something that just is at the moment.

Research shows that taking time to focus on things that you are grateful for increases your sense of social connection, meaning in life and subjective well-being[43].

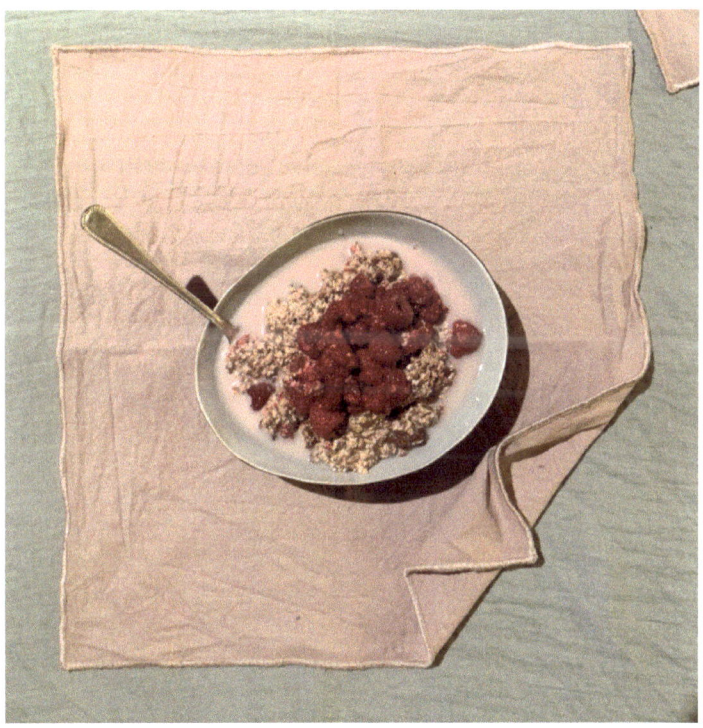

BREAKFAST – Raspberry & Chia Overnight Oats
[Serves 1, 10 minutes preparation]

Ingredients:

80g of oats	150ml water
Pinch of salt	1tsp apple cider vinegar
1tbsp chia seeds	60g frozen raspberries
1/2tbsp cocoa	Oat/hemp milk
1tbsp raisins	

Instructions:

Evening before:
1. Mix together all the dry ingredients in a bowl or a jar
2. Stir in the water and apple cider vinegar (make sure the chia seeds are well dispersed and everything is covered in water)
3. Top with the raspberries, cover and place in the fridge until tomorrow

In the morning before serving:
1. Remove the oats from the fridge a little before eating so they are not too cold
2. (If you have time you can heat them in a pot on the stove on a gentle heat)
3. Serve with a dash of oat milk (vary the amount based on your own preferences)

Try to sit down with your breakfast this morning and to eat it without doing anything else (like looking at your phone, watching TV, checking your work emails). I would encourage you to try and do this every morning this week if possible – but don't beat yourself up if it isn't, I know not everyone's schedule allows for this luxury.

Combining macronutrients

You will notice that most recipes in this book contain sources of carbohydrates, fats and proteins (have a look at the back of this book for some examples of each). This is because eating these three categories of 'macronutrients' together slows down the speed at which they are absorbed into your bloodstream, which means they provide a steady flow of energy or 'blood sugar' [44]. This reduces the likelihood of blood sugar spikes and dips, which both feel awful and can mimic the symptoms of anxiety and low mood (tearfulness, irritability, shakiness, dizziness) [6], [7].

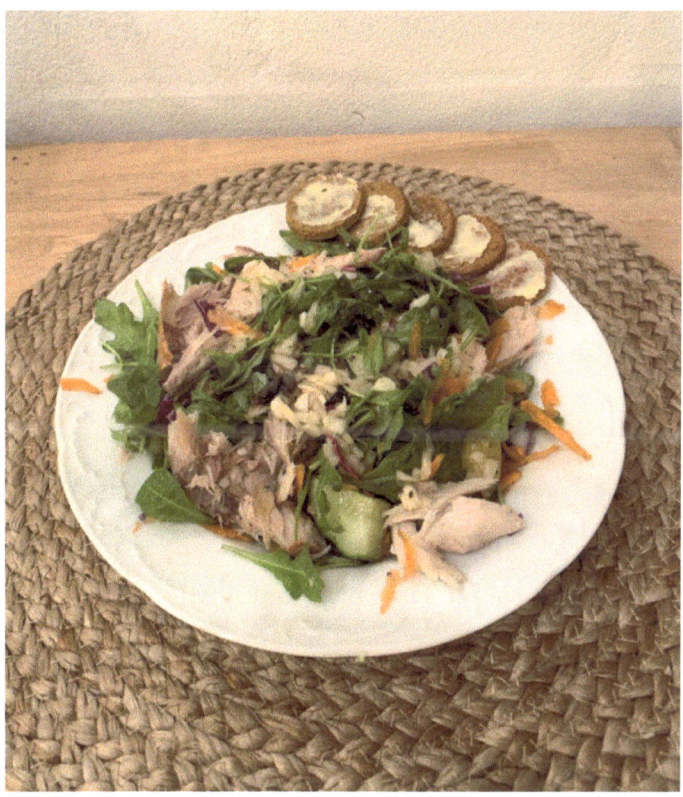

LUNCH – Salad Bowl
[Serves 1, 10-20 minutes preparation]

Ingredients:

Salad

80g of mixed salad leaves

1/4 cucumber, chopped

1/2 sprig of spring onion, chopped

1 carrot, grated

1 filet of smoked mackerel

2 tbsp pickled red cabbage

Optional topping: mixed seeds

Vinaigrette

5 tbsp olive oil

5 tbsp apple cider vinegar

5 tbsp water

1 tsp salt

1/2 tsp pepper

1 tsp dried mixed herbs

1 clove garlic, crushed and chopped

1 tsp honey

Serve with oatcakes or sourdough bread and butter

Instructions:
Evening before:
1. Prepare your ingredients
2. In a large enough bowl mix together all the salad ingredients, except the mackerel
3. Tear the mackerel into bite sized shreds and add to the salad
4. Cover or place in a container and store in the fridge until tomorrow
5. In another bowl mix together all the vinaigrette ingredients, store in a jar until tomorrow

The next day before serving:
1. Stir a tbsp or two of the vinaigrette through your salad, pour the remaining dressing into a jar and store in the fridge for later
2. You can sprinkle seeds over the salad if you like (these will be especially tasty if you very gently heat them in a dry pan for a few minutes)
3. Serve with oatcakes or sourdough and butter

Remember to try and sit down with your lunch and focus on what you are eating. Try to be outside if at all possible. Don't read, watch TV or look at your phone during lunch. If you can, eat lunch together with someone else.

Oily fish:
Oily fish is the main source of two types of omega-3 fatty acids: eicosapentaenoic acid (EPA) and docosahexaenoic acid (DHA) [45]. Omega-3 in general, and EPA and DHA in particular, are used by the body to regulate inflammation, blood sugar and weight[46]. The human brain is particularly rich in DHA and requires this for optimum functioning[46].

Over the last Century or so our diets and agricultural practices have changed dramatically, which has led to a lower intake of omega-3 and an increased intake of its counterpart – omega-6[46]. Omega-6 is found in most cultured plants, as well as factory, barn or farm-raised animals, whilst omega-3 is only really abundant in wild oily fish, pasture-raised animal products, and certain plants like rapeseed, chia and walnuts (although plant omega-3 needs to be converted to DHA and EPA before the body can use it) [46].

Although our bodies also need omega-6, it often has opposing functions to omega-3[46]. This means omega-6 is pro-inflammatory, whilst omega-3 down regulates inflammation[46]. Omega-6 is linked with worse blood sugar regulation, whilst omega-3 supports blood sugar regulation[46]. Omega-6 is linked with weight increases, whilst omega-3 may support weight loss[46].

Research has found decreased likelihood of depression in populations with a moderate oily fish intake [47]-[49], and some studies have found that omega-3 intake can have a positive impact on symptoms of low mood (particularly in women [47], overweight individuals [50] and individuals with higher levels of inflammation [51]). Omega-3 supplementation has also been linked with a reduction in symptoms of anxiety in a number of studies [52], [53].

SNACK – Sliced Banana
[Serves 1, 5 minutes preparation]

This week I would like you to practice not grazing. That means having a few hours between each time you eat (preferably 3-5 hours, but this will vary based on your body, so listen to how you feel).

I would also like you to practice not getting too hungry. This means that if it has only been an hour or two since you ate but you *are* hungry, then ignore my suggestion above and have a snack.

Nevertheless, ensure you eat all your snacks from a plate – and not straight out of a package. Each day I will give you a snack suggestion to help with this.

Ingredients:

1 banana

2tsp cocoa powder

1tbsp peanut butter

Instructions:

1. Peel your banana and slice it in half lengthwise
2. Cover each half with peanut butter and sprinkle with cocoa powder
3. Eat from a plate with a small spoon or fork

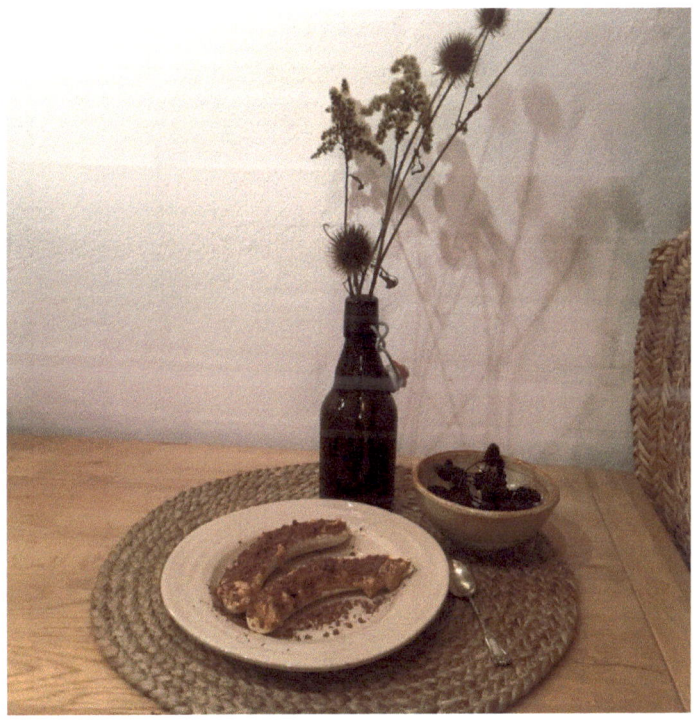

To make this snack portable, simply cut the banana into slices and place into a jar, top with cocoa and peanut butter – close and take with you. Remember a spoon!

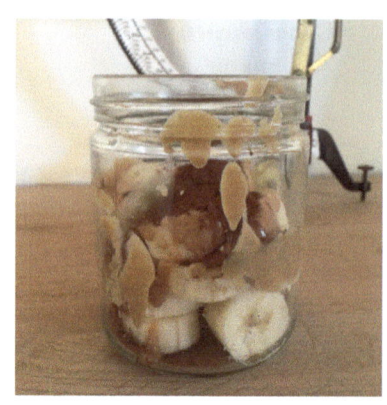

DINNER – Maharagwe (East African Bean Stew)
[Serves 2 – 15 minutes preparation, 45 minutes cooking]

Ingredients:

150g brown rice

1 cups water

1/2tsp salt

1 red onion, chopped

1 clove of garlic, crushed and chopped

1 tbsp of ginger, peeled and sliced

1 carrot, chopped

1 tin kidney beans

1 tin full fat coconut milk

2 handfuls of baby leaf spinach

50ml water + 1 cup water

Salt to taste (about 1/2 tsp)

(Optional) Avocado to serve

Instructions:

1. In a large enough pot heat up 50ml of water and begin preparing the onion, garlic, ginger and carrot - add each to the pot *as they are ready*
2. Open the tin of kidney beans and empty them into a sieve, rinse them carefully under cold water until there is no more foam - add to the pot
3. Shake the coconut milk well before opening and add **half** to the pot together with 1 cup of water
4. Add salt to taste and leave to simmer of medium heat, stirring occasionally
5. In another pot cook your rice by adding rice, 1 cups of water*, the remaining coconut milk and 1/2 tsp of salt
6. Cook the rice on high heat with the lid on until the water is boiling, then turn down the heat and remove the lid, allow to simmer for about 25 minutes or until tender (or follow package instructions)
7. When the rice is ready the stew will also be ready
8. Remove the stew from the heat and stir through the baby spinach
9. Serve with rice and avocado

*add more water if needed

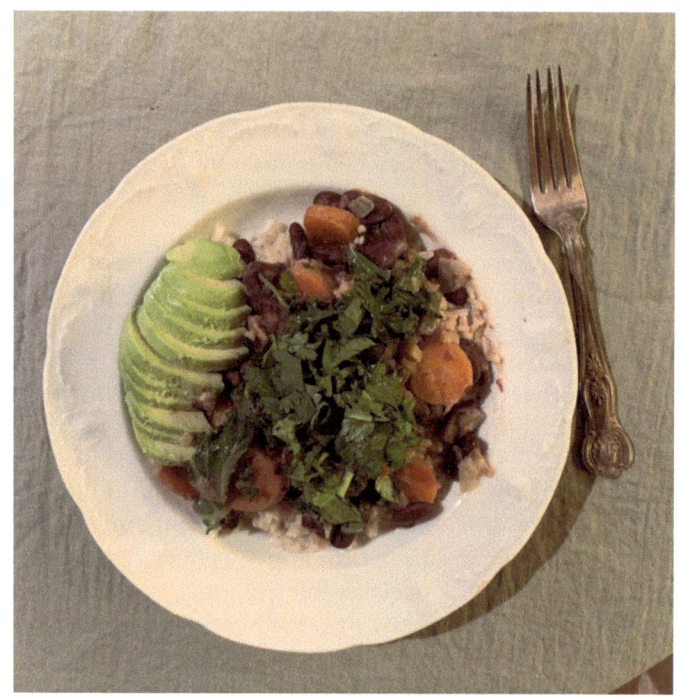

This recipe serves 2, so place the left overs in a container for your lunch tomorrow. Throughout this week the leftovers from your dinners are intended to be your lunch the next way. Remember to re-heat your food well.

PREPARATION FOR TOMORROW:
Before you go to bed tonight you need to do a little prep for tomorrow's breakfast. You will notice this section on most days of this 7-day challenge.

Go back to yesterday's breakfast recipe and follow the *'Evening before'* steps. Tomorrow morning you will do the remaining steps to have your breakfast.

Evening Reflection:

Well done for working through today. Whether you did all the steps or just a few of them – well done for doing it. Take some time before bed today to answer the following questions. You can write your answers down or just take a little time to think about them.

Is there anything you learned from today?

What part of today did you enjoy the most?

What did you do for others today?

What did you do for yourself today?

What (if anything) would you like to do differently tomorrow?

> "Today you are YOU.
> That is truer than true.
> There is no one alive
> Who is YOUER than you."
>
> -   Dr. Seuss

Good morning,

How are you feeling today? I'm glad you're back and reading on.

Before we start, take some time to think about what you are grateful for today.

Today I would like you to think about what it means to be you. So often we spend a lot of time and energy wishing we were different – more outgoing, less loud, did more of one thing and less of another, were taller, skinnier, bigger, smarter or more interesting, were calmer or kinder or funnier, had a more active job, had a less active job or had more friends.

Briefly check in with yourself if there are any repeated things you wish were different about you?

Read the text below and let it sink in. If you don't have time to read it right now, then take a picture on your phone and read it in your lunch break or read it on the commute to work or this evening in bed. But *really* read it. Let it sink in.

PRELUDE

"What if there is no need to change, no need to try to transform yourself into someone who is more compassionate, more present, more loving or wise?

How would this affect all the places in your life where you are endlessly trying to be better?

What if the task is simply to unfold, to become who you already are in your essential nature – gentle, compassionate, and capable of living fully and passionately present?

What if the question is not why am I so infrequently the person I really want to be, **but why do I so infrequently want to be the person I really am?**

How would this change what you think you have to learn?

What if becoming who and what we truly are happens not through thriving and trying but by recognising and receiving the people and places and practices that **offer us the warmth of encouragement we need to unfold?**

How would this shape the choices you make about how to spend today?"

Oriah Mountain Dreamer

What if there is no *need* to change.... what a wonderful notion. What if there is no n e e d to change.

You might be rolling your eyes at me right now. You might be thinking that I don't know you, that I would think differently if I met you. But bear with me. Today's challenge is a thought exercise I would like you to engage in every time you have thoughts about how you should be different, how you are inadequate or what you should or shouldn't be doing instead of what you actually *are* doing.

Challenge- Each time one of those thoughts comes up take a moment to answer the four questions below:

1. Is this a fact* or an opinion?
2. If it is a fact, is there anything I can do about it right now? (try to do it)
3. If it isn't a fact, does thinking about it change anything?
4. If a friend told me this thought about themselves, what would I say to them?

*Some rules about facts:
- facts are things that *have* happened, not things you think might happen
- facts are not subjective
- facts are not ambivalent
- facts are not based on your thoughts or opinions

TIP: answer the above four questions in writing instead of by simply thinking about them when negative thoughts come up throughout the day today.

A note on thoughts:
Have you spent much time thinking about what thoughts are? Where they come from, what they are made of? Most of us haven't. Most of us simply accept our thoughts as facts.

Did you know though that research shows that depressed individuals are more likely to have negative thoughts than when they aren't depressed or non-depressed individuals? That they are more likely to think a problem can't be solved[54]? That they are more likely to interpret situations negatively and remember negative events[54]? That anxious individuals are more likely to interpret situations as dangerous and less likely to think they can cope[54]? Although in the moment these negative thoughts feel like facts, in reality, they are a symptom of depression or anxiety, and believing the thoughts can feed the problem.

What is the difference between thinking: 'I am a failure' and 'I think I am a failure'? – Yes, you might feel like a failure, and you may think you are a failure, but does this make you a failure? Each time you think you are or aren't something try make sure you are clear on how you define that term. For example, what is a failure? Or if you think you can't cope, how do you define coping?

Learning to differentiate between what you think and what is a fact may be helpful in addressing low mood, anxiety and stress.

BREAKFAST- Overnight Oats
Hopefully your breakfast is ready and waiting for you.

Enjoy it! This breakfast is perfectly portable, so if you haven't got a lot of time simply take it with you and eat it on the bus or if necessary at the office (although I would always encourage you to try eating somewhere peaceful and not on the go, focused only on your food).

I am a big fan of focusing on the food we eat whilst we eat it, but I also know it can be really boring to eat alone. If this is you – try to listen to the radio or a podcast instead of scrolling on your phone or laptop or watching TV whilst you eat.

Whole-grains and the gut:
The recipes in this book often contain a source of whole-grains. These are the seeds of grain plants (like oats, wheat, rye or rice), which have not had their outer shell removed. This outer shell is often a rich source of vitamins, anti-oxidants, minerals and fibre [55]. By eating a variety of different types of whole-grains, instead of eating mostly wheat and rice, you increase the variety of nutrients and anti-oxidants you are consuming [56]. As mentioned at the beginning of the book, the greater the variety of fresh foods you consume the greater your variety of gut bacteria [32]. Although there is some conflicting evidence, research seems to indicate that eating more whole-grains can have a positive impact on the gut microbiome, inflammation and as a result the risk of developing chronic diseases [55].

Whole-grains might have an effect on inflammation and your gut microbiome in a relatively short time period. One study found that six weeks of eating a whole-grain rich diet as compared to a refined grain (where the outer seed shell has been removed) diet led to positive changes in gut and inflammatory markers [55]. Another study found that 6 weeks of a whole-grain diet as compared to refined grain diet led to a reduction in inflammatory markers, but no changes in the gut microbiome [57].

LUNCH- Leftover Maharagwe
I think the best way to make sure we eat a healthy, home-cooked lunch each day is to simply have leftovers from the day before! So today simply grab your leftover maharagwe, heat it up, top it with a spoonful or two of pickled cabbage and enjoy.

SNACK: Sourdough with Hummus & Cucumber
[Serves 1, 5 minutes preparation]

Ingredients:
1 slice of whole-grain sourdough bread

1 tbsp of hummus

8 slices of cucumber

Optional: butter

Salt and pepper to taste

Instructions:
1. Toast the bread
2. Spread with hummus (and butter if using)
3. Slice the cucumber and spread slices on top of the hummus
4. Sprinkle with salt and pepper to taste

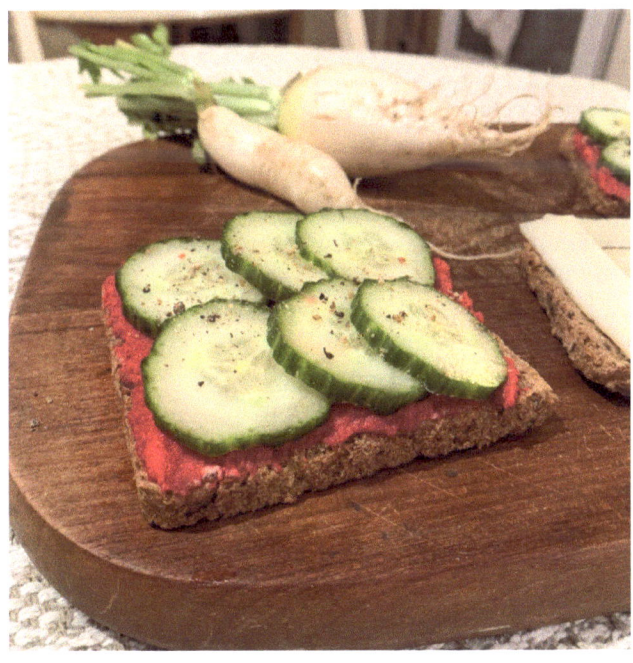

DINNER – Noodle Soup
[Serves 2 – 15 minutes preparation, 30 minutes cooking]

Ingredients:

200g chicken strips

2 cloves garlic, crushed and chopped

1 tbsp ginger, finely sliced

2 carrots, chopped

1 handful baby spinach

100g mushrooms sliced

1 tin coconut milk

700ml water1tsp salt

1 tsp olive oil

150g rice or soba noodles

2 sprigs of spring onion, chopped

Instructions:

1. In a large pot heat up the olive oil on a medium heat, add the chicken strips and cover with a lid
2. Prepare your garlic and ginger, add them to the chicken thighs
3. Flip the chicken strips onto their other side, pour over the coconut milk and allow to simmer
4. Prepare the carrots and mushrooms and add to the pot along with the salt and water
5. Allow to simmer for 20 minutes Add the noodles to the pot
6. Allow to cook for a further 5 minutes or until the noodles are soft
7. Stir through 1 handful of baby leaf spinach
8. Serve topped with chopped spring onion

Remember to put away a portion in a container or large jar for lunch tomorrow.

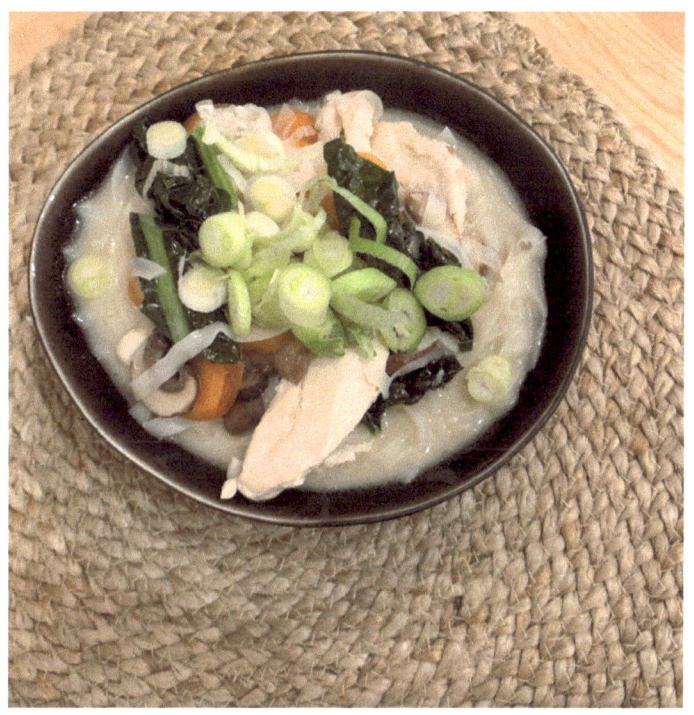

PREPARATION FOR TOMORROW:
Before you go to bed tonight you need to do a little prep for tomorrow's breakfast. You will notice this section on most days of this 7-day challenge.

Go back to yesterday's breakfast recipe and follow the *'Evening before'* steps. Tomorrow morning you will do the remaining steps to have your breakfast.

Evening Reflection:

Well done for working through today. Whether you did all the steps or just a few of them – well done for doing it. Take some time before bed today to answer the following questions. You can write your answers down or just take a little time to think about them.

Is there anything you learned from today?

What part of today did you enjoy the most?

What did you do for others today?

What did you do for yourself today?

What (if anything) would you like to do differently tomorrow?

DAY 3   MTWTFSS:

"God, grant me the serenity to accept the things I cannot
change,
the courage to change the things I can
and the wisdom to know the difference"
– Serenity Prayer

Good morning,

How did you sleep? How are you feeling about the
journey you are on this week with this book?

Before reading on take a moment to write down
something you are grateful for today:

Yesterday we started to think about our thoughts, how
they affect us and whether or not they are facts. I would
like you to do a little more thinking about thoughts
today.

The types of thoughts I would like you to think about
today are not the negative, present and past focused
thoughts we talked about yesterday, instead they are
negative future focused thoughts, otherwise known as
worries.

A note on worries:
A worry is a negative or catastrophic prediction of what the
future might bring. Often, we imagine the entire scenario of
how the future might look. When we are doing so in a worried
way we are normally imagining worst case scenarios.

As humans we actually worry a lot. In some ways it probably
makes us quite successful. It helps us understand the
consequences of events and actions, it prevents us from
engaging in risky behaviours, it helps us to respond to danger

signals. But worry is also exhausting - particularly when it is constant and doesn't lead to changes.

The benefits of worries I described just now come from identifying a problem, finding a solution and acting on that solution. When worry does not or *can* not lead to action it simply means we emotionally and mentally live through our fears over and over again.

Most worry comes from a desire for certainty. We would like to know for sure that nothing bad will happen, and we worry to try and find solutions in order to feel certain we can cope with the things that go wrong. The problem with this is that by worrying about it, by imagining the worst-case scenarios, we are actually living through the problems before they even happen. Sometimes we spend our entire lives mentally living worst-case scenarios that never actually happen.

The other problem is that each time we find a solution for our imagined problem our anxiety decreases a little bit – we feel better because we feel like we have found a solution. This temporary dip in anxiety teaches our brain that worrying reduces anxiety. So, your brain begins to throw more and more possible problems at you in an attempt to re-achieve that sense of temporarily reduced anxiety.

But how do you feel while you worry? *Anxious.* So, we worry more to feel less anxious, but the more we worry the more anxious we feel, and so we worry more.

What worries have been on your mind lately?
Challenge- At some point today take 15 minutes to do the following exercise with some of your most common worries.

On the left side of a piece of paper (or in your journal) write down all the worries that are *hypothetical,* these are worries about things that have not actually happened yet and may never happen. On the right side write down the worries that are *practical*, these are problems that are actually happening at the moment.

Example: If you are worrying that you may one day not be able to pay your rent because you may have unexpected costs, or you may lose your job, this is *hypothetical* because none of those things have happened yet. If you have lost your job and do not have enough money in your bank account to pay for your rent this month then the worry is *practical*, because it is a problem you have to deal with at the moment.

Hypothetical Worries:
When you have identified a hypothetical worry ask yourself the following questions:

1. Does worrying about this change anything?
2. How will I feel about this worry next week, next month, next year?
3. What would I say to a friend who had this same worry about themselves?

Practical Worries:
When you have identified a practical worry ask yourself the following questions:

1. [To double check it's **really** practical] Is this thing I am worried about **really** happening **right now?**
2. What can I do about this worry right now?
3. What can I do about it later?
4. Who can help me resolve this problem?

BREAKFAST - Overnight Oats
Enjoy your breakfast this morning – remember to try and focus on it while you eat it.

LUNCH - Leftover Noodle Soup
Remember to take your container of noodle soup with you today if you are not at home for lunch. Make sure to heat it up well before serving, and perhaps take a little left over chopped spring onion to sprinkle on top.

SNACK - Applesauce with Walnuts & Cinnamon
[Serves 1, 5 minutes preparation]

Ingredients:

100g apple sauce

Handful of walnuts

1/2 tsp of cinnamon

Optional: 2 tbsp live, natural yoghurt

Instructions:
1. Fill the apple sauce into a little bowl
2. Top with crushed walnuts and sprinkle with cinnamon
3. Add natural yoghurt on top if you wish

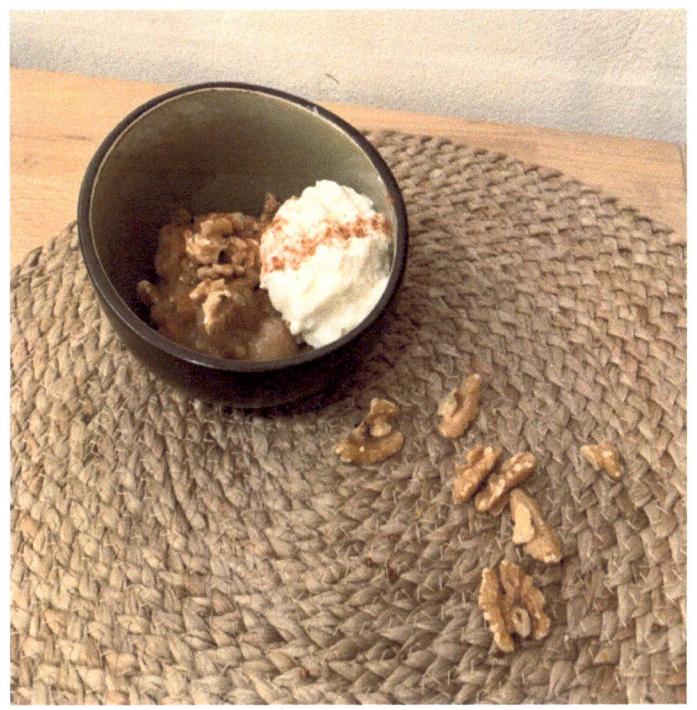

Challenge: If you have the time, I would like you to practice 'mindful eating' when you have your snack today. Follow the instructions below to do so:

- As you prepare your snack focus on what you can see, feel and smell. What colour does your bowl have? What colour do the apple sauce, the walnuts, the cinnamon have? What does the texture of each ingredient look like? What can you smell?
- Take your snack to a quiet place. Focus on how your footsteps feel on the ground as you walk there. Focus on how the air feels on your skin. Focus on what you can see around you.
- As you sit down to eat your snack focus on how it feels to sit. Are you sitting somewhere soft or hard?

How is your posture? What does your body feel like? Can you feel the sun on your skin?

- Then take a first spoonful, notice how it feels as the spoon enters the bowl, notice what it looks like as you move the spoon towards your mouth, notice whether the smells become more intense.
- Notice how the spoon feels in your mouth. What is the temperature like? How does the metal of the spoon feel? How does the apple sauce feel? How do the walnuts feel? How does the yoghurt feel?
- Notice how each component tastes, where do you taste it? Does the taste become more or less intense as you chew?
- Continue to notice these things with each spoonful you eat for as long as possible.

Before I give you today's dinner recipe I just want to talk a little bit about something called present moment focus – which actually plays an important role in learning to let go of hypothetical worries.

Present-moment Focus:

If you have already completed the worry exercise I gave you this morning you may have wondered what you are meant to do once you notice that some of your worries are hypothetical.

Hypothetical worries tend to be harder to let go of than practical worries. Once we notice a worry is practical we can make a plan for how to resolve the problem or ask for help in solving the problem, and then we tend to feel better. Once the problem is resolved we can let the worry go.

The real difficulties happen when we can do nothing about a problem. We can never do anything about hypothetical problems because those problems have not happened yet. Even worse- hypothetical worries tend to represent our worst fears, so we may feel unable to stop worrying about those things. For example, you may worry something really bad could happen to your child and you may feel not worrying about this would make you a bad parent. Really tricky practical worries may be like this – for example your partner may be terminally ill or your child may be doing badly in school despite your best efforts to help them get better.

I would argue that learning to let go of these worries does not mean you care less. It means you become better at coping with those situations that are out of your control. By worrying less about your child becoming ill you may be more able to enjoy your time with them. By focusing less energy on worrying about your partners terminal illness you may have more energy to invest into your final time with them.

Take a moment to reflect on how it feels to try and do something about something you can do nothing about.

Usually it is exhausting.

Present-moment Focus can provide an alternative response. This response involves acknowledging the problem or worry exists and acknowledging that you cannot do anything about it in this moment (perhaps because it has not happened or it is outside of your control). Then it requires re-focusing your attention to the present onto your current task (like you did in the mindful eating exercise).

You might have noticed that you don't worry as much when you are really engrossed in a conversation, task or movie. This is because we cannot think two things at the same time. By choosing to re-focus on the present moment instead of your worry you can learn to let those worries go that simply drain your energy and increase your anxiety.

Think of this as a new skill that you are learning. Just like learning to drive and shift gears- initially you will have to keep reminding yourself of what the different steps are and what you need to do, but over time it will become automatic and happen without you needing to think about it at all.

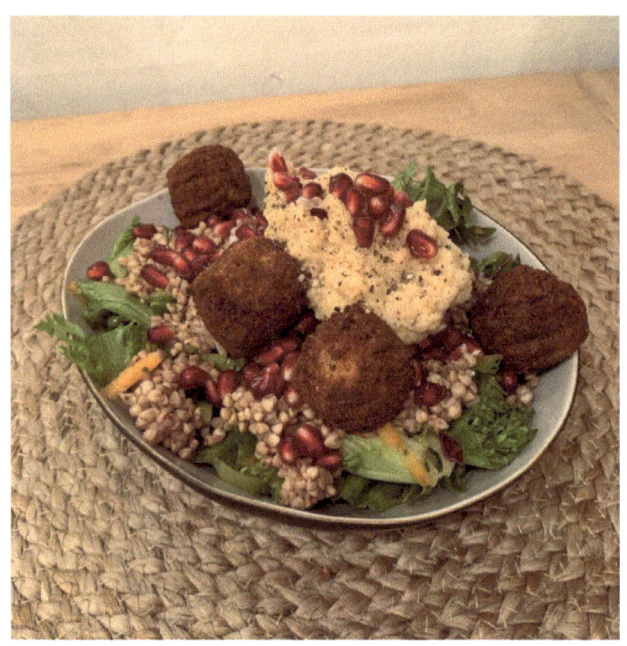

DINNER - Falafel, hummus & pomegranate salad
[Serves 2, 20 minutes preparation, 10 minutes cooking]

Ingredients:

125g mixed salad leaves

50g pomegranate seeds

1/2 cucumber, sliced

5 radishes, sliced

1 carrot, grated

1 sprig of spring onion, chopped

1 pack of falafels (at least 12)

2 tbsp of pickled cabbage

2 tbsp hummus

4 tbsp prepared salad dressing

80g quinoa

2 cups water

1 tsp salt

Instructions:
1. Place the quinoa in a pot and cover with water so that it is approximately 3cm under the water surface
2. Add 1 tsp salt and bring the water to a boil, then turn down to allow the quinoa to simmer for 10-15 minutes (until tender)
3. In the meantime, put the salad into a large bowl
4. Prepare the remaining fresh ingredients and add to the bowl
5. Top with falafels, pickled cabbage and pomegranate seeds
6. Stir through 4tbsp of the salad dressing you prepared on the first day
7. Once cooked, drain any remaining water from the quinoa and add to the bowl
8. Serve with a tbsp of hummus

As always, place the remaining food in a container for your lunch tomorrow, top with a tbsp of hummus.

EVENING PREPARATION:

You may have got used to the routine by now, but don't forget to prepare your breakfast for tomorrow. Below you will find a new overnight oats recipe – to mix things up a little bit.

BREAKFAST – Banana & Peanut Butter Overnight Oats

Ingredients:

60g of oats

Pinch of salt

1/2tbsp cocoa

1tbsp raisins

2tbsp peanut butter

150ml water

1tsp apple cider vinegar

1 banana, sliced

Oat/hemp milk

Instructions:

Evening before:
1. Mix together all the dry ingredients in a bowl/jar
2. Stir in the water and apple cider vinegar making sure everything is covered with water
3. Top with the sliced banana

In the morning before serving:
1. Remove the oats from the fridge a little before eating so they are not too cold
2. (If you have time you can heat them in a pot on the stove on a gentle heat)
3. Serve topped with peanut butter and a dash of oat milk (vary the amount based on your own preferences)

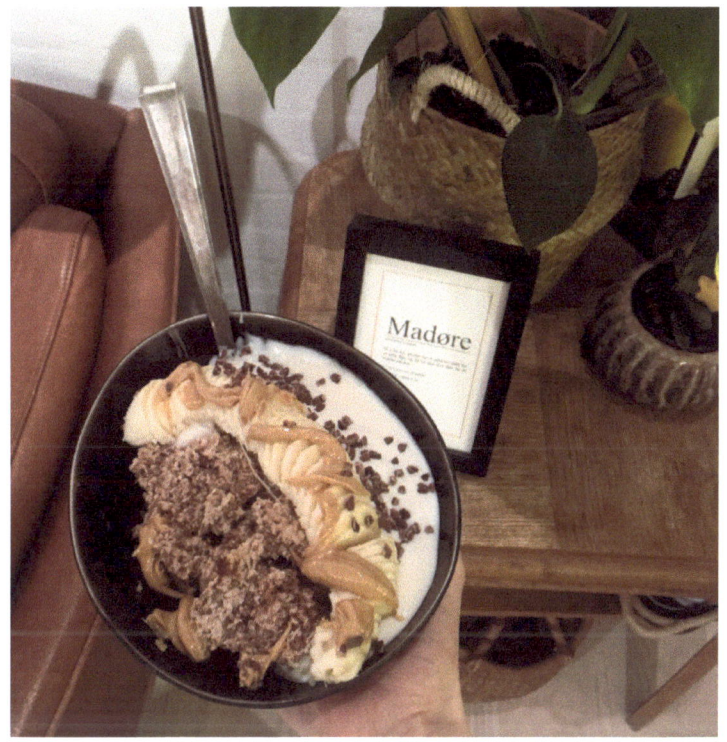

Evening Reflection:

I gave you quite a few things to do and think about today. I hope it didn't feel overwhelming. If you didn't manage to fit everything in take some time to think about when you might be able to do it instead. If you did do all the tasks, think about how you can start making things like the worry or thought questions you looked at in the last two days part of your routine. I encourage you to make present moment focus exercises part of your routine. Over the next couple of days, I will give you little prompts to do so.

Is there anything you learned from today?

What part of today did you enjoy the most?

What did you do for others today?

What did you do for yourself today?

What (if anything) would you like to do differently tomorrow?

I hope you have a cosy evening and sleep well tonight.

"fika
[fee-ka] – Swedish

(n.) a moment to slow down and
appreciate the good things in life"

Hello and good morning!

How are you today? Today you are half way through this
book, how does that feel?

Start this morning by writing down what you are grateful
for today.

I love the word fika. I wish it existed in all languages. The
fact that it doesn't just goes to show how little value we
place on slowing down in today's society.

Take a moment to write down what the good things in
life mean to you.

I think sometimes the problem with fika is that we don't
always know what the good things *are* for us. They are
different for everyone and change throughout life.

As children we're probably quite good at knowing – we
love being outside, getting our feet muddy, running until
our lungs burn, jumping into icy cold water, reading
scary stories in the dark with the light of just a torch,
eating candy as slowly as possible to make it last longer,
belly laughs, tickles, cuddles, watching insects or leaves,
feeling the wind or sun on our skin, enjoying the
sensation of being safe under an umbrella whilst the rain

pours down around us, building hide outs, play fighting, creating things like pressed flowers, drawings or poems.

But as adults? We don't always have time for those things. We don't always think they are important. We don't always remember how good they can feel.

Today take a moment to slow down and appreciate the good things in life.

I encourage you to do something outdoors today. If it is summery lie down in the grass somewhere and feel the sun on your face. If it is wintery take a brisk walk somewhere near trees. Do some stretching exercises outdoors. Go for a run or even better, go for a swim. If you can, jump into the water or go down a water slide.

Take time to notice what you are doing. Notice your surroundings. Notice the sounds. Notice the temperature and the feeling on your skin. Notice the smells. Take. T i m e .

In case today is a really busy day and you don't have time to take time for something 'big' like the things I have listed then do something small. Sit outside at lunch and listen to the birds. Walk part of the way home from work and notice people's gardens. Listen to music you love whilst you cook dinner and dance around the kitchen.

Write down what you will do today (and *really* do it – no matter how silly it feels):

Why exercise matters:
Research shows that during exercise muscle cells are able to take up blood sugar without insulin [5]. Regular aerobic exercise also increases cells' sensitivity to insulin, which can help to counter-act any insulin resistance that may have developed [5]. In fact, research shows that going for a simple 1-2 minute walk after a meal can help your body better regulate

the blood sugar rise from the food you just ate [58]. As I mentioned at the beginning of the retreat, worse blood sugar regulation can increase the likelihood of low mood or anxiety. Therefore, improving blood sugar regulation may have a positive effect on mood and anxiety.

Additionally, regular exercise or a physically active lifestyle may reduce inflammation – which, as you also read at the beginning of the retreat, may also have a positive impact on mood and stress [59].

BREAKFAST - Overnight Oats

I hope your breakfast is ready and waiting for you. Remember to savour it – perhaps it is even warm enough to sit outside with it? Under a tree?

LUNCH - Leftover Falafel Salad
Don't forget to take your lunch with you today!

SNACK - Sourdough, Manchego Cheese & Radishes
[Serves 1, 5 minutes preparation]

Ingredients:

1 slice whole-grain sourdough bread

30g Manchego cheese, sliced

Handful of radishes

Optional: butter

Instructions:
1. Toast the bread
2. Spread with butter if using
3. Top with sliced Manchego cheese and serve with radishes

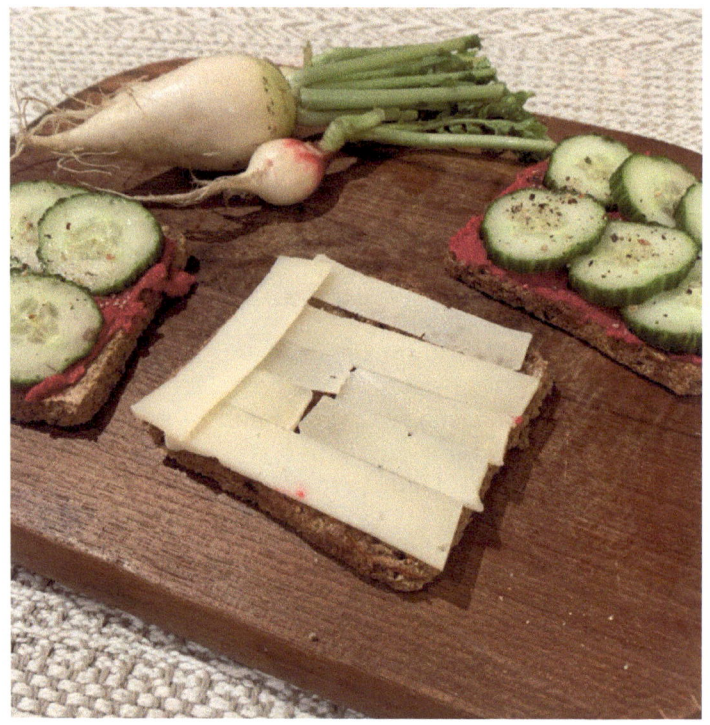

If you haven't had a chance for fika by the time you have your snack, then why not take it outside (weather allowing) and make some time to enjoy it slowly.

Below you will find your dinner recipe for today. As always, place the remaining food in a container for your lunch tomorrow. In case there is more than you need you can keep the rest in the freezer for another week.

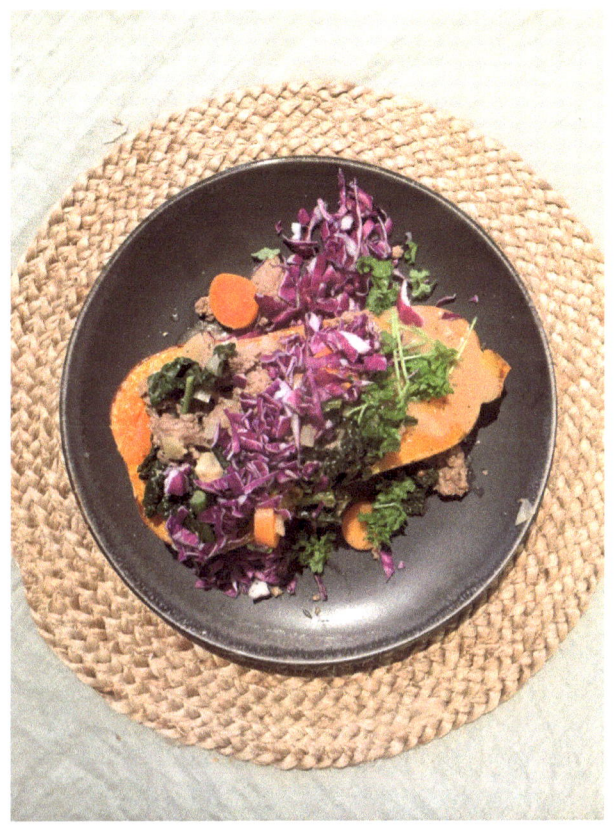

DINNER – Butternut Squash with Ragout
[Serves 2, 15 minutes preparation, 30 minutes cooking]

Ingredients:

1 medium butternut squash, halved length-wise and de-seeded

1 onion, chopped

1 clove garlic, crushed and chopped

50g baby leaf spinach

1 carrot, finely sliced (width wise)

1 tbsp chopped parsley

1/2 tin coconut milk **(skim off the cream and place in the fridge - you will use this on day 6)**

Juice of 1/2 a lime

200g beef mince

3tsp olive oil

Salt and pepper to taste

2 tbsp pickled red cabbage

Instructions:
1. Pre-heat the oven to 180 degrees C
2. Prepare your squash, rub the cut surfaces with 2tsp olive oil, salt and pepper
3. Place on a lined baking tray, then put in the oven and allow to bake for 30-40 minutes
4. After 10 minutes heat 1 tsp olive oil in a pan and then add the minced beef, allow to brown, stirring from time to time
5. In the mean-time prepare the onion and garlic and add to the pan along with 1/2 tin coconut milk
6. Prepare the carrot and add to the pan
7. Season with salt and pepper as well as any other herbs/spices you wish and have on hand (e.g. cumin, paprika or mixed herbs) and lime juice
8. Allow to simmer, stirring occasionally until all ingredients have cooked through
9. The ragout should be ready around the same time as the butternut squash
10. Remove the pan from the heat and stir through the spinach
11. Serve by topping half of the butternut squash with a generous serving of ragout, 1 tbsp pickled cabbage and sprinkle with parsley

PREPARATION FOR TOMORROW:
Don't forget to prepare your breakfast for tomorrow. Go back to page 58 for the recipe.

Evening Reflection:
Take some time to answer the questions below:

How do you think you could make more space for fika in your everyday life?

Is there anything you learned from today?

What part of today did you enjoy the most?

What did you do for others today?

What did you do for yourself today?

What (if anything) would you like to do differently

tomorrow?

"you can't go back and change the beginning, but you
can start where you are and change the ending."
-    C.S. Lewis

Good morning,

How are you today? Only 3 days left of this journal now!

Start the day by writing down something you are grateful
for.

Today's challenge may feel a little tricky. It's also a lot of
reading, so if you haven't got time to do it right now (I
would guess it will take about 20 minutes) schedule a
time to do it later today.

I want to talk about regret and forgiveness. Regret about
past decisions, actions or situations, and forgiveness of
our own or others' actions. Research shows us that
greater levels of regret and lower levels of forgiveness are
linked with a greater likelihood of depression and
anxiety[60]–[63]. Learning to manage regret and grudges
or hurts differently may have a positive impact on your
wellbeing[61], [62].

Forgiveness and Regret

Some researchers argue that forgiveness is a character trait, in that some people are actually more disposed to forgiving than others [4]. This includes forgiving yourself as well as forgiving others. If you struggle with forgiveness, it might be a trait - but this does not mean you can't change the way you think about and practice forgiveness.

The less we forgive, the more regret we experience. And so regret and forgiveness go hand in hand.

It is important to recognise that forgiving is not the same as condoning[64]. By forgiving something that was done to you, or something you yourself have done, you are not necessarily saying that the action was justified. Clinging on to initially justified emotions (such as anger at being mis-treated) can have negative emotional consequences, and so forgiving allows you to let go of such emotions when they linger long after the event [64].

The below definition of forgiveness expresses this notion beautifully:

"A willingness to abandon one's right to resentment, negative judgment, and indifferent behaviour to one who unjustly injured us, while fostering the undeserved qualities of compassion, generosity and even love toward him or her" [65]

You are often absolutely justified in feeling anger or resentment. The question is simply - do these justified feelings help you meet the need those emotions are expressing?

With regard to regret, research shows that low mood increases our likelihood of feeling regret [66]. This indicates, that regardless of actual outcomes, when you feel low you are more likely to regret your decisions or the outcomes of situations. To me, this highlights again the subjective and unreliable nature of our thoughts and feelings – remember from day 2: thoughts are not facts. Feelings of regret do not necessarily mean that alternative decisions or outcomes would have been better. I would actually argue that regret is often based on the belief that we know things would have been different or better if we or someone else had acted differently. But we don't know that.

We can't know that. We are simply imagining an alternative reality and believing it would have been true if only we or they had done something differently.

You may be thinking 'That's all well and good, but forgiveness and letting go of regrets are two things I would like to do but have no idea *how* to do'. Fair enough.

One study defines forgiveness as: "a voluntary coping process involving offering, feeling, or seeking a change from negative to positive cognitions, behaviours, and affect toward a transgressor"[67].

Let's break that down. "A voluntary coping process" – that means we have to *choose* to forgive ourselves or the transgressor. You have probably heard that before right? But *how* to choose and *why* to choose?

Let's start with the why. Take a moment to write down how regret and holding on to past hurts makes you feel (perhaps think about a specific example). How does it feel physically? How does it feel emotionally?

How does it affect how you behave (towards yourself or the other person)?

Does regret or holding on change anything about what happened in the past?

Thinking about regret specifically, do you *know for a fact* that a different action or decision would have led to a different (and especially better) outcome?

Holding the above three things in mind; do regret or not forgiving serve you in any way? If yes, how?

You may be thinking that regret and none forgiveness protect you from future mistakes or future hurt. But remember – forgiveness does not mean you condone that action. You can still learn from something without holding onto the negative feelings.

Now let's look at the *how*.

"Seeking a change from negative to positive cognitions, behaviours, and affect toward a transgressor"[67].

Look back at the question on how the regret or lack of forgiveness affects how you behave. This might include thoughts, things you say or don't say and things you do or don't do.

If you no longer regretted that action, or if you were no longer holding onto the things you haven't forgiven, how might you behave differently?

Remember – forgiving is not condoning. Forgiveness does not necessarily mean you need to become best friends with someone who has hurt you. It may simply mean no longer talking about everything they have done to you at every opportunity. Forgiving yourself for missing an important work deadline does not mean you think it is okay to miss deadlines and you are going to keep missing them in future. It may simply mean taking note when you start mentally beating yourself up for missing that deadline and re-directing your thoughts to some of the questions above, or those we went through about thoughts and worries on days 2 and 3. Or you might want to think about what you have learned from that situation and how you will do things differently in future.

I do have one bit of bad news though. Doing this once won't make much difference. In the words of Martin Luther King Jr:

"Forgiveness is not an occasional act, it is a constant attitude"
– Martin Luther King Jr

So after that long introduction, here is today's challenge: Think of something you have not forgiven, this may be a regret about something you did or a hurt about something someone else did, write it down now in your journal if you can.

What change will you make in terms of how you think about this situation or behave with regard to it in order to make a first step towards forgiveness?

BREAKFAST – Overnight Oats
You're breakfast is hopefully almost ready and waiting for you.

LUNCH – Leftover Roast Squash & Ragout
Enjoy your lunch of leftovers today and remember to heat the food well before eating.

SNACK – Juicy Dates with Peanut Butter and Cocoa
[Serves 1, 5 minutes preparation]

Instructions:

4 Dates

1 tbsp peanut butter

1 tsp cocoa powder

Instructions:

1. Halve the dates and take out the seeds
2. Fill each half with peanut butter
3. Sprinkle with cocoa powder
4. Serve and enjoy one half at a time

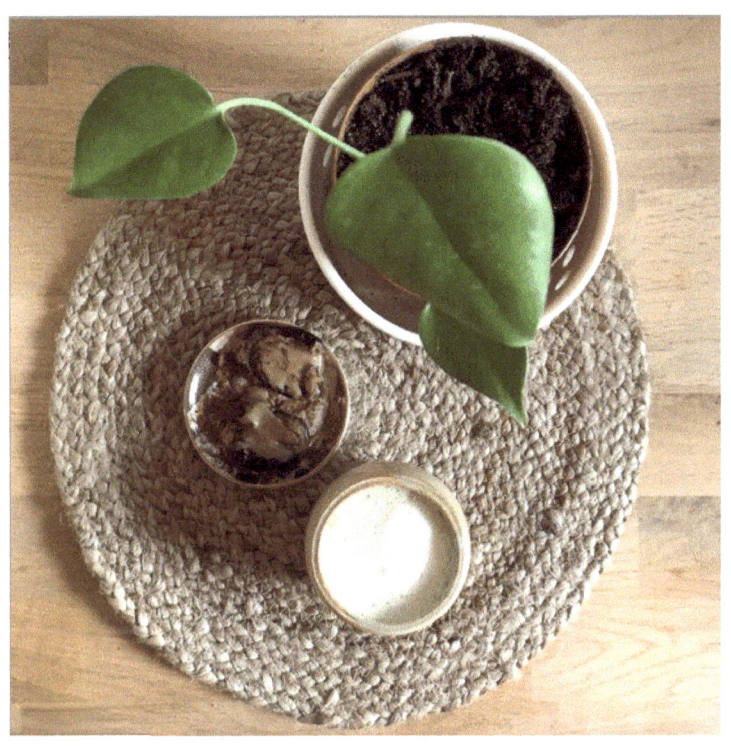

DINNER – Green Pasta
[Serves 1, 5 minutes preparation, 15 minutes cooking]

Ingredients:

1 onion, chopped

2 cloves garlic, crushed and chopped

Juice of 1/2 lemon

100g frozen broccoli florets

100g frozen peas

2tbsp olive oil + more to drizzle

1/2 cup water + 1 pot water

120g Edamame/soy/chickpea pasta

1.5 tsp salt + salt and pepper to taste

Optional: chopped parsley

Instructions:
1. Prepare your onion and garlic
2. In a large pan heat up 1tbsp of olive oil, add the onion and garlic and allow to brown for 2 minutes
3. In the mean-time bring a pot of water to the boil, add the pasta and 1tsp salt, cook according to instructions on the pasta package
4. Add the frozen broccoli, peas, 1/2 cup of water and 1/2 tsp salt to the pan and allow to simmer for about 8 minutes
5. Add the lemon juice to the pan with vegetables, stir through, then remove from the heat once broccoli is tender
6. Strain the pasta once tender and stir through the vegetables
7. Serve drizzled with extra olive oil, salt, pepper and parsley

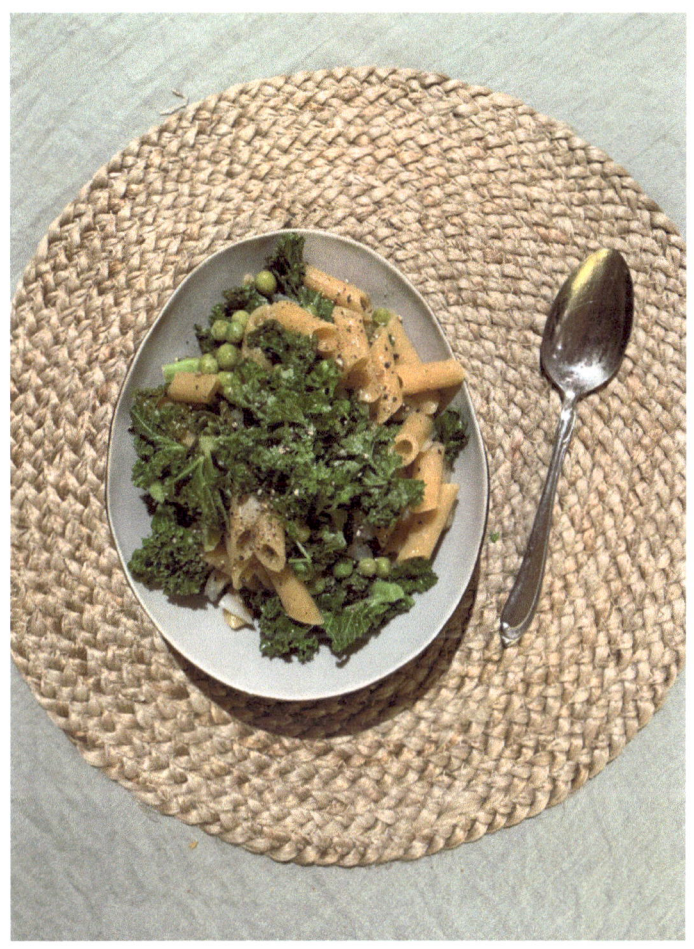

PREPARATION FOR TOMORROW

Today you don't need to do any prep for your breakfast, because I am hoping you will have time to make it from scratch tomorrow. This is of course assuming that you have more time on the weekends – which may not be the case. *If you need to, you can prepare the pancakes this evening and simply heat them up in the morning by popping them in the oven for 5-10 minutes at 180 degrees C. You will find the recipe on page 79.*

Evening reflection

I hope you have been thinking about regret and forgiveness today. If you haven't had a chance to read today's challenge yet, do it now ☺ If you have, take some time to reflect on today using the questions below.

Is there anything you learned from today?

What part of today did you enjoy the most?

What did you do for others today?

What did you do for yourself today?

What (if anything) would you like to do differently

tomorrow?

"The most effective way to do something, is to do it."
- Amelia Earhart

Hello and good morning!

Welcome back! Well done for checking in each day.

As always, take a moment to write down something you are grateful for before getting started with your day.

What do you think of today's quote?
It actually annoys me.

Of course the most effective way to do something is to do it. But what if I don't know how? Or I don't feel able to? Or I have so much other stuff to do I can't find the peace of mind to do that thing I'm not doing?

Procrastination
Did you know that depression and anxiety both increase and are exacerbated by procrastination [1]? When we are anxious or low (or stressed) we are much more likely to think we won't be good at something, won't be able to do it, won't be able to find a solution or we won't enjoy it [2]. Other times we just don't see the point. No wonder some things feel impossible to do.

But research also shows that doing more (routine things like the laundry, sociable things like calling a friend, important things like paying a bill, physical things like doing some exercise) are really beneficial in improving the way we feel [3],[4]. Overcoming procrastination can be a key to achieving this.
Write down an activity that you have been avoiding (**just one thing**). It might be a chore like putting away the clean laundry or opening a letter or going through your emails. It might be responding to friends and family, by

replying to a message for example. It might be something physical, like going to a gym class, doing a morning run or trying out a home yoga video. It might be starting a new book. It might be anything at all – what comes to your mind first?

Today I challenge you to do that activity for just 2-5 minutes.

Set a timer and fold laundry and put it away until the timer goes off. Open and read emails until the timer goes off.

 Go for a five-minute run (don't stop yourself by thinking 'If I only do five minutes there is no point' – I know that's what just came to your mind).

Do it!

If you *want to* continue after five minutes you absolutely can. But the goal is just to do five minutes.

From now on, each morning, set yourself an activity (that you normally avoid) that you will do for five minutes that day.

BREAKFAST – Fluffy Pancakes
[Serves 1, 5 minutes preparation, 15 minutes cooking]

Ingredients:

100g buckwheat flour

2 tbsp linseeds

1/2 tsp baking powder

Dash of salt

Dash of ground cardamom (optional)

150ml water

Butter or olive oil for frying

Frozen berries

Banana

Apple sauce

Dark chocolate

Peanut butter

Live, natural yoghurt

Seeds

Honey

Toppings (choose your favourites):

Instructions:
1. In a large bowl mix together all the dry ingredients
2. Whisk in 150ml water with a fork
3. Heat oil in a frying pan and add 1 large tbsp of batter per pancake once the pan is hot
4. Turn the heat down slightly (to medium)
5. Flip the pancakes once they start to have a slightly dry appearance on top
6. Remove from the pan once lightly golden on both sides, repeat with the remaining batter
7. Serve with suggested toppings or whatever else you please.

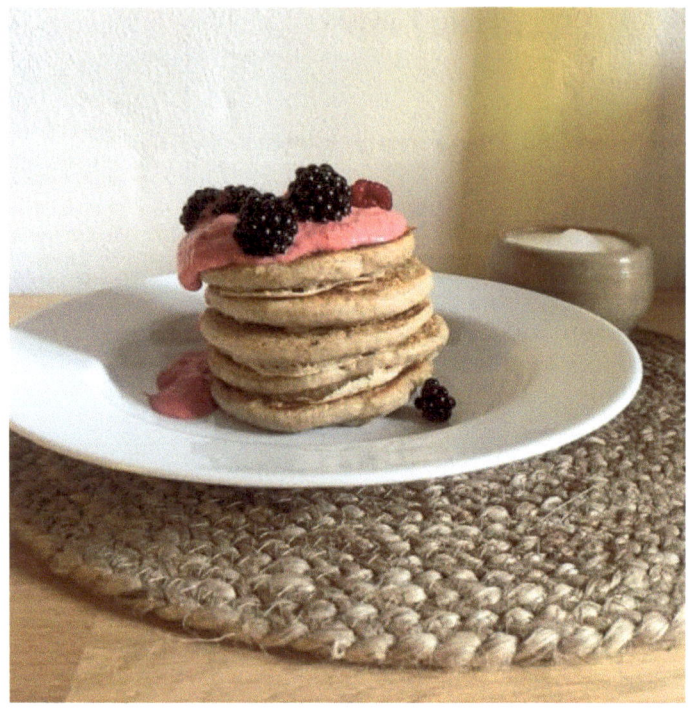

If you have time this morning – head to the kitchen now and nourish yourself with some delicious pancakes. If you don't then I hope you prepared your pancakes last night – in which case all you need to do is warm them up (in the oven or a pan) and top them with whatever you like.

Enjoy!

Fermented (or probiotic) foods

You may have noticed that quite a few of the recipes include fermented or live foods. For example, pickled cabbage or live yoghurt. The reason for this is that these foods often contain what I call 'friendly bacteria' for your gut. These little guys are necessary to regulate your immune system, to help your body digest nutrients, to create nutrients that your body can absorb and even to create the neurotransmitters (or brain chemicals) that help us to feel motivated, calm and happy [5], [6]. Not only that, fermented foods also tend to enhance the beneficial nutritional properties of the food – for example, they may contain far more bioavailable phytochemicals than the none fermented version of the food [7], [6].

By including fermented, unpasteurised foods in your diet you are increasing the chances of your gut being full of friendly guys (rather than unfriendly guys who can contribute to inflammation, digestive discomfort and mood swings). Certain fermented foods like sauerkraut or kimchi have the added benefit of being full of fibre – in other words food for the friendly guys [5]. Without food they don't last long in your gut!

Research suggests that this can lead to improvements in both mood and anxiety [8], [6]!

A little side note: the unfriendly guys thrive off sugar and refined carbohydrates [9]. Take a moment to think about which guys you are feeding with your normal diet?

Tip: Increase fibre and probiotic foods slowly, overloading your digestive system with too many new guys or too much fibre can cause digestive discomfort!

LUNCH – Green Pasta Leftovers

Enjoy your leftovers today. If today is Saturday – why not go outside to enjoy it? Or meet with a friend?

SNACK – Raspberry and Coconut Ice-cream
[Serves 1, 5 minutes preparation, 30 minutes waiting (optional)]

Ingredients:

5 tbsp Coconut cream in fridge (from day 4)

80g frozen raspberries

Toppings:

1 or 2 squares dark chocolate- broken into bits

Handful of crushed walnuts

Instructions:
1. Place all the ingredients (except the toppings) into a blender and blend until smooth*
2. Serve immediately topped with walnuts and dark chocolate, or place in the freezer for 15-30 minutes to increase firmness first

*You can also use a hand blender for step 1. Alternatively place the ingredients in a bowl and whip with a whisk or fork until combined - this will not be as smooth as it would be from a blender.

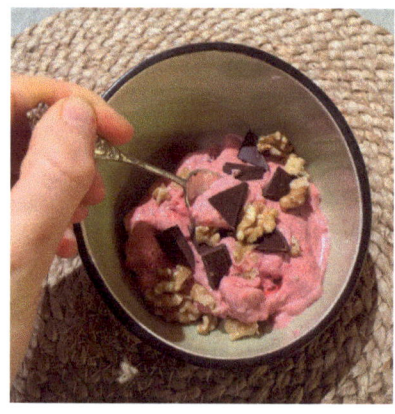

Have you completed your challenge yet? If not take five minutes to do so now.

DINNER – Baked Sweet Potato with Tuna Salad
[Serves 2, 10 minutes preparation, 40 minutes cooking]

Ingredients:

2 medium sweet potatoes

1/2 cucumber, cut into small cubes

1 sprig of spring onion, chopped

1 tbsp parsley, chopped

3 radishes, sliced

1 carrot, grated

160g tinned tuna

2 tbsp prepared vinaigrette

2 tbsp red cabbage (optional)

1 tbsp olive oil

Salt and pepper to taste

Instructions:
1. Pre-heat the oven to 180 degrees C
2. Whilst it is heating up scrub your sweet potatoes clean under running water, but do not peel them
3. Cut the sweet potatoes in half and drizzle the cut side with olive oil and sprinkle with salt
4. Place on a lined baking tray (cut side up) and bake for about 30 minutes or until soft and slightly caramelised around the edges
5. Whilst they are baking prepare your vegetables and mix them together with the (strained) tuna in a bowl
6. Stir in the vinaigrette and red cabbage, add more salt and pepper if needed
7. Once the potatoes are ready take them out of the oven and serve topped with tuna salad

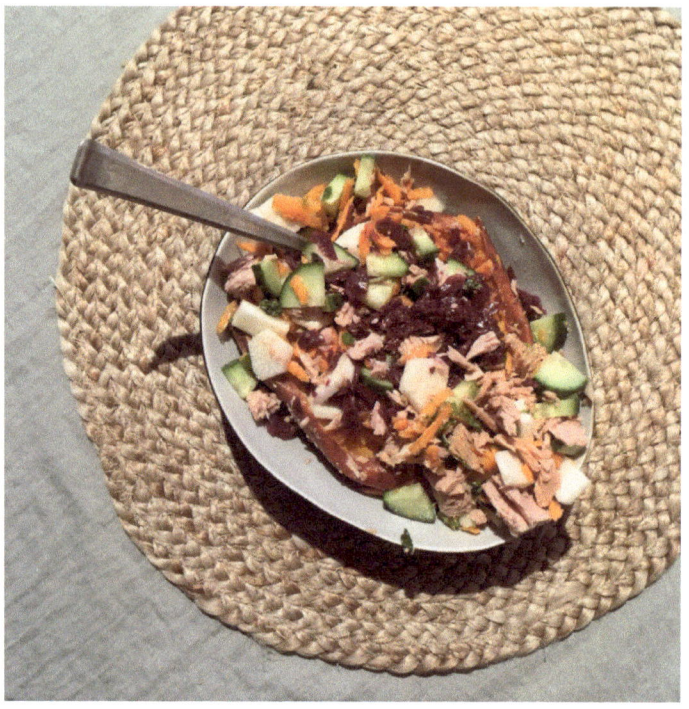

Tip: Tomorrow's snack requires a bit of baking. In case you prefer to do it now you can find the recipe below.

If you don't have time to prepare breakfast from scratch tomorrow, you can also use these oat-y flapjacks as a breakfast instead of the recipe you will find tomorrow. Simply cut yourself a slightly bigger slice and top with live yoghurt and fruits.

SNACK – Oat Flapjacks
[Serves 6, 15 minutes preparation, 15 minutes baking]

Ingredients:

2 bananas, mashed

75g butter, room temperature

2 eggs

2 tsp apple cider vinegar

1 tsp cinnamon

1/2 tsp ground cardamom

1 tsp salt

50g dark chocolate

2 tbsp chia seeds

50g crushed walnuts

140g oats

Instructions:
1. Pre-heat the oven to 200 degrees C (top and bottom heat)
2. Chop the butter into small chunks, then mash together with the bananas using a fork
3. Whisk in the eggs
4. Add the vinegar, cinnamon, cardamom and salt, mix well
5. Break the chocolate into small pieces and stir through the mix
6. Mix in the chia seeds, crushed walnuts and oats
7. Line a baking tray with baking paper and spread the batter out over the tray until it is about 1cm thick (make any shape you like)
8. Bake at 200 degrees C for 15 minutes
9. Take it out when it is lightly golden and cut into 10-12 pieces

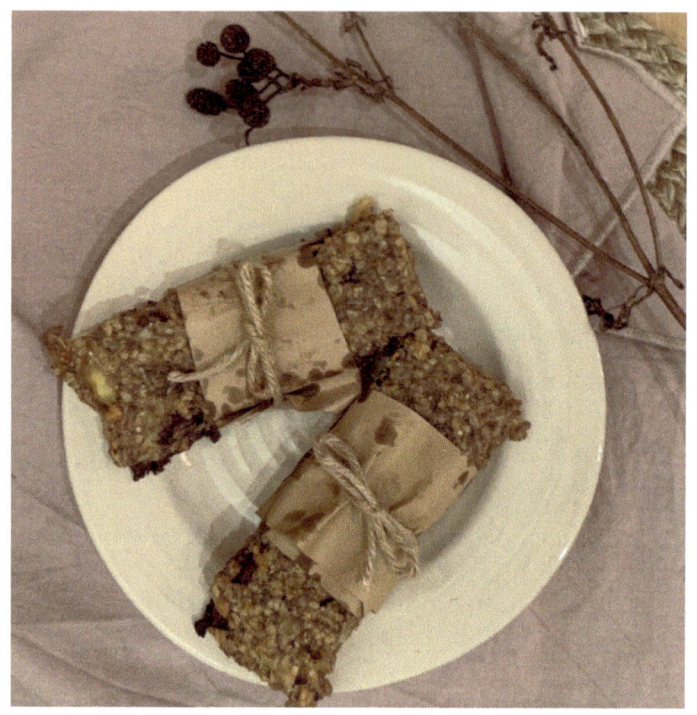

Evening reflection:
Look at you! Only one day left of the retreat! Well done for getting to this point. Take some time now to reflect on how it feels.

Is there anything you learned from today?

What part of today did you enjoy the most?

What did you do for others today?

What did you do for yourself today?

What (if anything) would you like to do differently

tomorrow?

DAY 7   MTWTFSS:

> "To live is the rarest thing in the world. Most people
> exist, that is all."
> -   Oscar Wilde

Good morning,

you are here again, on the last day of this journal. Well
done, for everything you have done so far. You may not
have made all the recipes, read all the parts or done all
the challenges.

But having come this far – you have done some things. I
can't say enough how proud you should be of this. This
retreat requires you to take time out of your daily
routine, to do things differently, to write things down
and to reflect. That isn't easy. So well done.

Once again, write down some things you are grateful for
today.

This retreat has been about taking care of yourself in the
best possible way right now, regardless of what is going
on around you.

Part of taking care of ourselves is spending time,
thoughts and energy on the things that bring us joy.

That means finding those *"people and places and practices
that offer us the warmth and encouragement we need to
unfold"* (Oriah Mountain Dreamer).

We can spend a lot of time perfecting a healthy diet, a
regular exercise routine, completing projects at work or
keeping our home clean and tidy. The thing is though –
these things on their own will not change anything
unless they bring you joy, meaning and purpose.

We can do a lot of things because we should. In fact – in today's society we do most things because we feel we should. Social media, capitalism and the idea that we should always be moving forwards – onwards and upwards to the next goal, all keep us moving, searching, feeling like we should be doing more.

Today, try to notice every "should" and "shouldn't" that come into your mind.

Notice it, and then try to ask yourself "What do I want to do?" instead.

Perhaps follow that up with: "Why do I want to do that?"

For example, this evening when you come home you might think:

"I should tidy up the kitchen".

Notice that should. Notice how it makes you feel.

Then check in with yourself what you want. Do you want to be surrounded by clean and calm surroundings? If so, perhaps you *want* to tidy the kitchen?

Or do you want to get outside because you have been sitting inside all day? Then go for a walk. Or do you want to sit down on the sofa and listen to music for a while because you have been rushed off your feet all day? Then sit down. Listen to what you want and why you want it.

Then make an intentional choice about how you spend your time. *Don't simply listen to that should ... just because you think you should.*

BREAKFAST – Omelette
[Serves 1, 10 minutes preparation time, 10 minutes cooking]

Ingredients:

2 eggs*

1 tbsp parsley, chopped

50g baby leaf spinach

150g mushrooms, sliced

Juice of 1/2 lime

1 sprig of spring onion, chopped

Salt and pepper to taste

1 tbsp butter

Optional: 1 Avocado

Sourdough bread/oatcakes and butter to serve

*See alternative ingredients for vegan omelette

Instructions:
1. Prepare all your ingredients
2. In a bowl whisk the eggs and spring onion, season with salt and pepper to taste
3. In a pan heat up 1/2 tbsp of butter on a medium heat and pour in the egg mix, allowing it to spread across the pan
4. In another pan heat up the remaining butter and add the sliced mushrooms, allow to brown for about 5 minutes, season with salt and pepper to taste
5. Once the egg mix has a bubbly, dry texture on top (after about 2-3 minutes), use a spatula to flip it and cook on the other side
6. Stir the spinach and lime juice through the mushrooms after about 5 minutes Slide the omelette onto a plate, top with the mushrooms and fold in half
7. Serve with avocado, bread and butter, sprinkle with chopped parsley

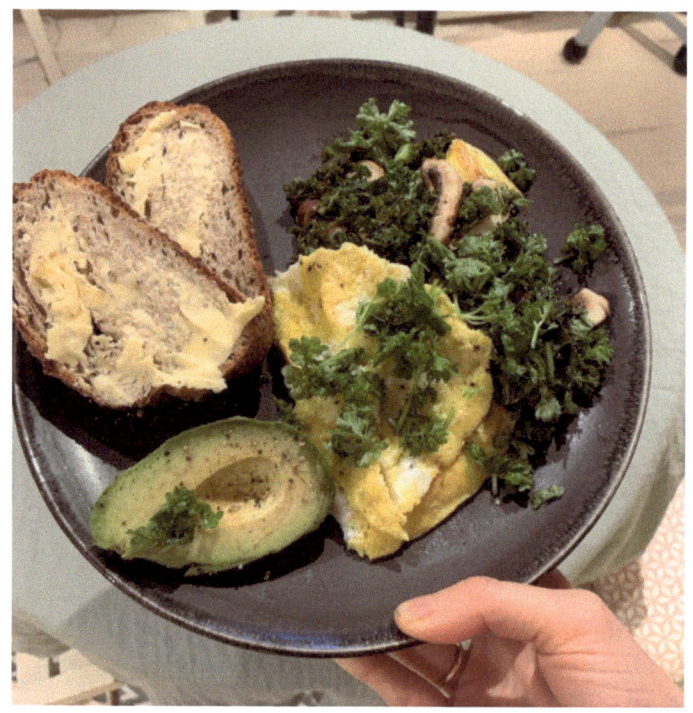

LUNCH – Left over Sweet Potato & Tuna Salad

Enjoy your left-over sweet potato and tuna salad for lunch today. I would recommend re-heating the sweet potato, it is much better warm than cold.

SNACK – Oat Flapjack

If you didn't prepare this yesterday, then go ahead and do so at some point today. You will find the recipe on page 85.

Cut into 10-12 pieces and enjoy topped with live yoghurt or peanut butter.

Pause for a minute

Have shoulds been on your mind today?

Think back to fika, how it felt to make time for the good things. Not filling the day with shoulds and shouldn'ts.

How can you take this principle and apply it to the broader aspects of your life? To your daily purpose?

Take a moment to write down all the things you do because you should in a typical day.

Now take a moment to write down all the things you do because they bring you joy, a sense of connection, a sense of achievement or a sense of purpose.

How can you make more time for the second category of things? How can you re-connect with the 'why' behind the things you do because you feel like you should do them?

Perhaps you exercise because you feel like you should. You don't eat a second biscuit because you feel like you shouldn't. You text your mum because you feel like you should.

Those are all good things you are doing. But if you are just doing them because you feel that you should they are unlikely to be as fulfilling as they could be.

Take an item from your should list, and write down all the reasons why you do it. If you can't come up with any good reasons why, then re-evaluate if you want to keep investing energy into it. If you do come up with good reasons – does the 'should' turn into an 'I want to'?

Should item:

Reasons why I do it:

What do I want to do with this activity going forwards:

DINNER – Mustard-y Broccoli Rice
[Serves 2, 10 minutes preparation, 30 minutes cooking]

You can serve this with some salad seasoned with the dressing you made at the beginning of the week if you wish.

Remember to put away half of this meal in a container for your lunch tomorrow.

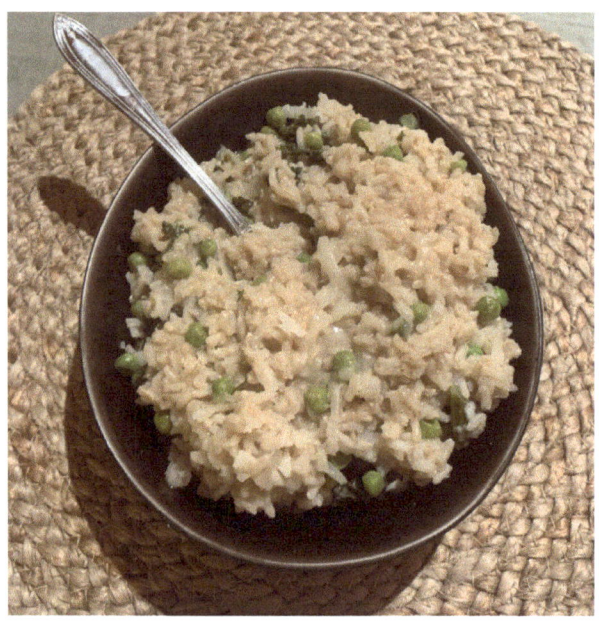

Ingredients:

1 tsp olive oil

1 onion, chopped

2 cloves garlic, crushed and chopped

180g brown rice

3 cups water

1 tsp salt

100g frozen peas

100g frozen broccoli

2 tbsp mustard

2 tbsp grated Manchego cheese

1 tbsp butter

Instructions:

1. Prepare your onion and garlic, put into a pot together with 1tsp olive oil and brown for 2-5 minutes
2. Stir regularly, then add the rice, tsp of salt and 3 cups of water
3. Cover and allow to simmer on low-medium heat for 20 minutes, stirring occasionally
4. Add the broccoli, peas and mustard to the rice, add more water if needed to prevent the rice from sticking to the base of the pot
5. Allow to simmer for a further 10 minutes
6. Remove the pot from the heat when the rice is fully cooked and most of the water has evaporated
7. Stir through the Manchego cheese and butter before serving
8. You can serve this with some salad and left over vinaigrette (optional)

Evening Reflection:

Today was your last day of your journal. Of course, you can keep coming back to the recipes, the meal plan, the challenges and anything else that you have found helpful. Finishing these seven days doesn't mean everything goes back to how it was before you started this book – or at least I hope it doesn't.

What were your favourite things about this retreat?

What did you find the most difficult?

What would you like to continue doing going forwards?

How will you do it?

How have things changed for you over the past week?

What is the most important thing you learned this week?

How are you going to start your day tomorrow?

You've done it. You have completed the retreat. I hope you found the experience helpful and nourishing. That it has given you some knowledge and skills that you can carry forward into your everyday life. There is an empty meal plan, as well as an activity schedule available at the back of this book. You can use these to think about how you will carry on your favourite things going forwards.

But for now – good night, I hope you sleep well.

How to use the Meal Plan and Shopping List

Important reminder: Whilst I am a nutritional therapist, I am not *your* nutritional therapist. That means this meal plan and the accompanying shopping list are not created exactly for *your specific needs*. They are provided as guidance only and you should adjust them so that they fit your needs. If you know you do not tolerate certain foods well then please replace those recipes with something else. *Always* **speak to your medical practitioner before making any significant changes to your diet.**

You will notice that the breakfast during the week is always the same – this is simply because feedback showed that making a different breakfast every day of the week can feel stressful.

You will also notice that all lunches except the Monday lunch are 'left overs'. This is because I know that making both dinner and lunch from scratch can feel incredibly overwhelming. By cooking extra at dinner, you automatically ensure that you have a wholesome, home cooked lunch ready for you the next day.

Notice the * next to your Monday lunch. This is because that is the only day where you don't eat left overs, and this is because I am assuming you will start on a Monday. If for any reason you do not start on a Monday, then you will need to shift the lunches to match the day you start.

The plan is written for one person and therefore recipes at breakfast always serve 1 and recipes at dinner serve 2 (to ensure you have left overs for the next day). If you are cooking for more people than this, you will need to multiply the ingredients by the number of people that you are. Note the section in the shopping list of ingredients that *you do not need to multiply* if you are cooking for more than one person.

The * next to ingredients like butter indicates that if you are vegan or vegetarian you will need to choose an alternative ingredient.

After the shopping list you will find a list of common ingredients, as well as alternatives.

For example, you may have noticed on the shopping list that you need buckwheat flour. However, you may not be able to find that in your local store. Head over to the alternatives lust and check under *Flours*. Here you will find a number of flours you can buy instead.

Similarly, if you are vegan or vegetarian and need an alternative for the tuna in the recipe for Saturday, simply head over to the alternatives album and check under *Protein*.

Meal Plan

	MON	TUE	WED	THU	FRI	SAT	SUN
BREAKFAST	Overnight Oats	Overnight Oats	Overnight Oats	Overnight Oats	Overnight Oats	Fluffy Pancakes	Omelette
LUNCH	Salad Bowl	Left Overs	Left Overs	Left Overs	Left Overs	Left Overs	Left Overs
DINNER	Maharagwe (Rice & Beans)	Noodle Soup	Falafel & Hummus Salad	Butternut Squash with Ragout	Green Pasta	Baked Sweet Potato & Tuna Salad	Mustard-y Broccoli Rice
SNACK	Sliced Banana	Sourdough with Hummus & Cucumber	Apple Sauce with walnuts & cinnamon	Sourdough with Manchego cheese and Radishes	Juicy Dates with Peanut Butter	Raspberry ice cream	Oat Flapjack

Blank Meal Plan

	BREAKFAST	LUNCH	DINNER	SNACK
MON				
TUE				
WED				
THU				
FRI				
SAT				
SUN				

Shopping List

Fridge:

Eggs* - 4

Unsalted butter* - 250g

Manchego cheese* - 75g

Live natural yoghurt
(dairy or coconut) - 250
to 400g

Hummus - 100g

Smoked mackerel - 1
filet*

Beef mince - 200g*

Chicken strips - 200g*

Pack of falafels - at least
10 pieces

Baby spinach - 250g

Mixed salad- 205g

Frozen broccoli - 200g

Frozen peas - 200g

Spring onion - 5 to 6

Parsley - 1 bunch

Cucumbers - 2

Carrots - 7 to 8

Mushrooms - 250g

Radishes - about 13

(Red) Onions - 4

Garlic - 2 heads

Ginger - 1 large piece

Sweet potatoes - 2
medium sized

Butternut
squash/pumpkin - 1

Avocado - 2

Bananas - 5 or 6

Lemon - 1

Lime - 1

Pomegranate seeds - 50g

Frozen raspberries -
500g

Pantry:

Quinoa - 80g

Oats - 500g

Brown rice - 330g

Buckwheat flour - 100g

Soba noodles or rice
noodles - 150g

Edamame or chickpea
pasta - 120g

Oatcakes - 1 package of
at least 12

Sourdough bread - (6
slices, you can freeze the
remaining bread)

Chia seeds - 100g

Linseeds - 20g

Mixed seeds, optional - 75g

Walnuts - 100g

Raisins - 100g

Fresh dates - 4

Apple sauce - 200g

Dark chocolate (above 70% cocoa) - 100g

Coconut milk - 3 tins

Tinned tuna in olive oil or water - 160g*

Kidney beans - 1 tin

Pickled red cabbage - 1 jar

Items you do not need to multiply if you are cooking for more than on person:

Jar of peanut butter (you will need 6 tbsp of this)

Jar of honey (you will need a few tsp of this)*

Jar of mustard (you will need a few tsp of this)

A bottle of extra virgin olive oil - you will use this for cooking and salad dressing

A bottle of apple cider vinegar - you will use this for salad dressing

A pack each of:

Salt

Pepper

Mixed dried herbs

Cinnamon

Cardamom (optional)

Baking powder (you will need 1/2tsp this week)

Cocoa powder (you will need 5tbsp this week)

Oat/almond/soy milk - 1l

Alternatives

Greens:

Salads

Mixed salad leaves
Rocket
Baby spinach
Iceberg lettuce
Endive
Little gem lettuce
Watercress
Rainbow chard
Mustard greens
Romaine
Radicchio

Herbs

Parsley
Coriander
Basil
Chives
Dill
Rosemary
Oregano

Vegetables

Cucumber
Peas
Green beans
Asparagus
Broccoli
Bok choy
Kale
Zucchini
Cabbage
Mangetouts
Sugar snap peas
Avocado
Brussels sprouts
Celery
Green olives
Okra
White cabbage
Fennel
Romanesco

Coloured Vegetables:

Tomato
Radish
Carrot
Aubergine
Purple cabbage

Sweetcorn
Yellow, orange or red peppers
Beetroot
Bamboo shoots

Kalamata olives (not black olives)

Cauliflower

Coloured vegetables to use as a carbohydrate rich side

Sweet potato

Celeriac

Parsnip

Butternut squash

Pumpkin

Cassava root

Yam

Jerusalem artichoke

Potato

Fruits:

Blackberries

Blueberries

Raspberries

Pomegranate

Strawberries

Banana

Apple

Orange

Khaki

Mango

Pineapple

Grains:

Quinoa

Brown rice

Red rice

Wild rice

Buckwheat groats

Spelt grains

Pearl barley

Millet grains

Sorghum grains

Oats

Whole-wheat pasta/noodles

Chickpea/lentil pasta

Rice/soba noodles

Flours:

Oat flour (you can make your own by pulsing oats in a blender until they turn to flour)

Buckwheat flour

Whole-grain wheat flour

Whole-grain spelt flour

Gram (chickpea) flour/besan

Protein:

Meat (uncooked)

Chicken

Beef

Minced meat

Lamb

Venison

Pheasant

Boar

Pork

Sausage

Offal like liver, kidneys or heart (try to ensure these are organic)

Meat (cooked)

Pre-cooked chicken breast

Prosciutto

Ham

Roast beef

Speck

Liver paté

Seafood

Any fresh fish or seafood (to cook)

Smoked mackerel

Smoked salmon

Smoked trout

Tinned mackerel (choose tinned fish in water, olive oil or brine)

Tinned (wild) salmon

Tinned sardines

Tinned tuna

Tinned crab meat

Dairy and eggs

Egg

For vegan omelette use gram (chickpea) flour

Feta (not salad cheese)

Manchego cheese

Roquefort

Parmesan

Pecorino cheese

Plant

Seeds (chia, linseeds, pumpkin, sunflower)

Nuts (walnuts, brazil nuts, almonds, hazelnuts, macadamia nuts, cashew nuts, pecans)

Legumes (chickpeas, peanuts, lentils, beans - e.g. kidney beans, black beans, broad beans, cannellini beans, soybeans, peas)

Hummus

Tofu

Tempeh

Falafels

Fats:
Olive oil
Avocado oil
Butter
Ghee

Other:
You can switch Sourdough Bread for
Gluten-free bread

Oatcakes

Rice-cakes

Crisp-bread

Seeded whole-meal bread

Sweet potato or another starchy vegetable

You can switch Pickled Red Cabbage for
Sauerkraut

Pickled beetroot

Raw, finely sliced cabbage

You can switch Peanut Butter for
Almond butter

Cashew butter

Hazelnut butter

Pumpkin seed butter

Sunflower seed butter

Bibliography

[1]   N. Marty, M. Dallaporta, and B. Thorens, "Brain Glucose Sensing, Counterregulation, and Energy Homeostasis," *Physiology*, vol. 22, no. 4, pp. 241–251, Aug. 2007.

[2]   G. Pocock, *Human Physiology*, 5th ed. Oxford: Oxford University Press, 2017.

[3]   N. M. Sanders *et al.*, "The selective serotonin reuptake inhibitor sertraline enhances counterregulatory responses to hypoglycemia," *Am. J. Physiol. Metab.*, vol. 294, no. 5, pp. E853–E860, May 2008.

[4]   M. Webb *et al.*, "The association between depressive symptoms and insulin resistance, inflammation and adiposity in men and women," *PLoS One*, vol. 12, no. 11, p. e0187448, Nov. 2017.

[5]   L. Sherwood, *Human Physiology: From Cells to Systems*. Cengage Learning, 2015.

[6]   NHS, "Hyperglycaemia (high blood sugar) - NHS," 2018. [Online]. Available: https://www.nhs.uk/conditions/high-blood-sugar-hyperglycaemia/. [Accessed: 26-Jun-2019].

[7]   NHS, "Low blood sugar (hypoglycaemia) - NHS," 2017. [Online]. Available: https://www.nhs.uk/conditions/low-blood-sugar-hypoglycaemia/. [Accessed: 26-Jun-2019].

[8]   E. Dror *et al.*, "Postprandial macrophage-derived IL-1β stimulates insulin, and both synergistically promote glucose disposal and inflammation," *Nat. Immunol.*, vol. 18, no. 3, pp. 283–292, Mar. 2017.

[9]   G. Rajkowska and C. A. Stockmeier, "Astrocyte Pathology in Major Depressive Disorder: Insights from Human Postmortem Brain Tissue."

[10]   J. E. Beilharz, J. Maniam, and M. J. Morris, "Short-term exposure to a diet high in fat and sugar, or liquid sugar, selectively impairs hippocampal-

dependent memory, with differential impacts on inflammation," *Behav. Brain Res.*, vol. 306, pp. 1–7, Jun. 2016.

[11]   L. N. Masi *et al.*, "Combination of a high-fat diet with sweetened condensed milk exacerbates inflammation and insulin resistance induced by each separately in mice," *Sci. Rep.*, vol. 7, no. 1, p. 3937, Dec. 2017.

[12]   I. Kang, J. C. Espín, T. P. Carr, F. A. Tomás-Barberán, and S. Chung, "Raspberry seed flour attenuates high-sucrose diet-mediated hepatic stress and adipose tissue inflammation," *J. Nutr. Biochem.*, vol. 32, pp. 64–72, Jun. 2016.

[13]   P. Kumar Jena, B. Prajapati, P. Kumar Mishra, and S. Seshadri, "Influence of Gut Microbiota on Inflammation and Pathogenesis of Sugar Rich Diet Induced Diabetes," 2016.

[14]   R. Strawbridge, D. Arnone, A. Danese, A. Papadopoulos, A. Herane Vives, and A. J. Cleare, "Inflammation and clinical response to treatment in depression: A meta-analysis," *Eur. Neuropsychopharmacol.*, vol. 25, no. 10, pp. 1532–1543, Oct. 2015.

[15]   S. E. Holmes *et al.*, "Elevated Translocator Protein in Anterior Cingulate in Major Depression and a Role for Inflammation in Suicidal Thinking: A Positron Emission Tomography Study," *Biol. Psychiatry*, vol. 83, no. 1, pp. 61–69, Jan. 2018.

[16]   F. Lamers, Y. Milaneschi, J. H. Smit, R. A. Schoevers, G. Wittenberg, and B. W. J. H. Penninx, "Longitudinal Association Between Depression and Inflammatory Markers: Results From the Netherlands Study of Depression and Anxiety," *Biol. Psychiatry*, vol. 85, no. 10, pp. 829–837, May 2019.

[17]   R. Yirmiya, N. Rimmerman, and R. Reshef, "Depression as a Microglial Disease," *Trends Neurosci.*, vol. 38, no. 10, pp. 637–658, Oct. 2015.

[18]   M. R. Dolsen, A. D. Crosswell, and A. A. Prather, "Links Between Stress, Sleep, and Inflammation: Are there Sex Differences?," *Curr. Psychiatry Rep.*, vol. 21, no. 2, p. 8, Feb. 2019.

[19]   A. A. Prather, N. Vogelzangs, and B. W. J. H. Penninx, "Sleep duration, insomnia, and markers of systemic inflammation: Results from the Netherlands Study of Depression and Anxiety (NESDA)," *J. Psychiatr. Res.*, vol. 60, pp. 95–102, Jan. 2015.

[20]   V. Michopoulos, A. Powers, C. F. Gillespie, K. J. Ressler, and T. Jovanovic, "Inflammation in Fear- and Anxiety-Based Disorders: PTSD, GAD, and Beyond," *Neuropsychopharmacology*, vol. 42, no. 1, pp. 254–270, Jan. 2017.

[21]   J. Gaines *et al.*, "Inflammation mediates the association between visceral adiposity and obstructive sleep apnea in adolescents," *Am. J. Physiol. Metab.*, vol. 311, no. 5, pp. E851–E858, Nov. 2016.

[22]   M. Lucas *et al.*, "Inflammatory dietary pattern and risk of depression among women," *Brain. Behav. Immun.*, vol. 36, pp. 46–53, Feb. 2014.

[23]   C. M. Phillips, N. Shivappa, J. R. Hébert, and I. J. Perry, "Dietary inflammatory index and mental health: A cross-sectional analysis of the relationship with depressive symptoms, anxiety and well-being in adults," *Clin. Nutr.*, vol. 37, no. 5, pp. 1485–1491, Oct. 2018.

[24]   S. Dutheil, K. T. Ota, E. S. Wohleb, K. Rasmussen, and R. S. Duman, "High-Fat Diet Induced Anxiety and Anhedonia: Impact on Brain Homeostasis and Inflammation," *Neuropsychopharmacology*, vol. 41, no. 7, pp. 1874–1887, Jun. 2016.

[25]   M. Peet and D. F. Horrobin, "A Dose-Ranging Study of the Effects of Ethyl-Eicosapentaenoate in Patients With Ongoing Depression Despite Apparently Adequate Treatment With Standard

Drugs," *Arch. Gen. Psychiatry*, vol. 59, no. 10, p. 913, Oct. 2002.

[26] B. Nemets, Z. Stahl, and R. H. Belmaker, "Addition of Omega-3 Fatty Acid to Maintenance Medication Treatment for Recurrent Unipolar Depressive Disorder," *Am. J. Psychiatry*, vol. 159, no. 3, pp. 477–479, Mar. 2002.

[27] H. Khodabandehloo, S. Gorgani-Firuzjaee, G. Panahi, and R. Meshkani, "Molecular and cellular mechanisms linking inflammation to insulin resistance and β-cell dysfunction," *Transl. Res.*, vol. 167, no. 1, pp. 228–256, Jan. 2016.

[28] A. H. Miller and C. L. Raison, "The role of inflammation in depression: from evolutionary imperative to modern treatment target," *Nat. Rev. Immunol.*, vol. 16, no. 1, pp. 22–34, Jan. 2016.

[29] C. L. Raison *et al.*, "A Randomized Controlled Trial of the Tumor Necrosis Factor Antagonist Infliximab for Treatment-Resistant Depression," *JAMA Psychiatry*, vol. 70, no. 1, p. 31, Jan. 2013.

[30] L. Galland, "Diet and Inflammation," *Nutr. Clin. Pract.*, vol. 25, no. 6, pp. 634–640, Dec. 2010.

[31] MyNewGut, "The Microbiome's influence on energy balance, brain development, diet-related diseases and behaviour," 2018.

[32] T. G. Dinan *et al.*, "Feeding melancholic microbes: MyNewGut recommendations on diet and mood," *Clin. Nutr.*, 2018.

[33] J. A. Foster, L. Rinaman, and J. F. Cryan, "Stress & the gut-brain axis: Regulation by the microbiome," *Neurobiol. Stress*, vol. 7, pp. 124–136, Dec. 2017.

[34] K. Rea, T. G. Dinan, and J. F. Cryan, "The microbiome: A key regulator of stress and neuroinflammation," *Neurobiol. Stress*, vol. 4, pp. 23–33, Oct. 2016.

[35] P. M. Munyaka, E. Khafipour, and J. E. Ghia, "External influence of early childhood

establishment of gut microbiota and subsequent health implications," *Frontiers in Pediatrics*, vol. 2, no. OCT. Frontiers Media S.A., 01-Oct-2014.

[36] T. A. Jenkins, J. C. D. Nguyen, K. E. Polglaze, and P. P. Bertrand, "Influence of tryptophan and serotonin on mood and cognition with a possible role of the gut-brain axis," *Nutrients*, vol. 8, no. 1. MDPI AG, 20-Jan-2016.

[37] J. M. Yano *et al.*, "Indigenous bacteria from the gut microbiota regulate host serotonin biosynthesis," *Cell*, vol. 161, no. 2, pp. 264–276, Apr. 2015.

[38] T. G. Dinan *et al.*, "Feeding melancholic microbes: MyNewGut recommendations on diet and mood.," *Clin. Nutr.*, vol. 0, no. 0, Nov. 2018.

[39] L. Costantini *et al.*, "Impact of Omega-3 Fatty Acids on the Gut Microbiota," *Int. J. Mol. Sci.*, vol. 18, no. 12, p. 2645, Dec. 2017.

[40] A. Nanri *et al.*, "Dietary patterns and depressive symptoms among Japanese men and women," *Eur. J. Clin. Nutr.*, vol. 64, no. 8, pp. 832–839, Aug. 2010.

[41] I. Jeffery and P. O'Toole, "Diet-Microbiota Interactions and Their Implications for Healthy Living," *Nutrients*, vol. 5, no. 1, pp. 234–252, Jan. 2013.

[42] E. D. Sonnenburg and J. L. Sonnenburg, "Starving our microbial self: The deleterious consequences of a diet deficient in microbiota-accessible carbohydrates," *Cell Metabolism*, vol. 20, no. 5. Cell Press, pp. 779–786, 04-Nov-2014.

[43] K. Y.-H. Liao and C.-Y. Weng, "Gratefulness and subjective well-being: Social connectedness and presence of meaning as mediators.," *J. Couns. Psychol.*, vol. 65, no. 3, pp. 383–393, Apr. 2018.

[44] D. Jakubowicz *et al.*, "High-energy breakfast based on whey protein reduces body weight, postprandial glycemia and HbA1C in Type 2 diabetes," *J. Nutr. Biochem.*, vol. 49, pp. 1–7, Nov.

2017.

[45]   National Institutes for Health, "Omega-3 Fatty Acids," 2019.

[46]   A. Simopoulos, Simopoulos, and A. P., "An Increase in the Omega-6/Omega-3 Fatty Acid Ratio Increases the Risk for Obesity," *Nutrients*, vol. 8, no. 3, p. 128, Mar. 2016.

[47]   Y. Yang and Y. Je, "Fish consumption and depression in Korean adults: the Korea National Health and Nutrition Examination Survey, 2013–2015," *Eur. J. Clin. Nutr.*, vol. 72, no. 8, pp. 1142–1149, Aug. 2018.

[48]   A. Sánchez-Villegas *et al.*, "Mediterranean dietary pattern and depression: the PREDIMED randomized trial," *BMC Med.*, vol. 11, no. 1, p. 208, Dec. 2013.

[49]   M. Berger *et al.*, "Cross-sectional association of seafood consumption, polyunsaturated fatty acids and depressive symptoms in two Torres Strait communities," *Nutr. Neurosci.*, pp. 1–10, Aug. 2018.

[50]   S. A. Keshavarz *et al.*, "Omega-3 supplementation effects on body weight and depression among dieter women with co-morbidity of depression and obesity compared with the placebo: A randomized clinical trial," *Clin. Nutr. ESPEN*, vol. 25, pp. 37–43, Jun. 2018.

[51]   M. H. Rapaport *et al.*, "Inflammation as a predictive biomarker for response to omega-3 fatty acids in major depressive disorder: a proof-of-concept study," *Mol. Psychiatry*, vol. 21, no. 1, pp. 71–79, Jan. 2016.

[52]   K.-P. Su *et al.*, "Association of Use of Omega-3 Polyunsaturated Fatty Acids With Changes in Severity of Anxiety Symptoms," *JAMA Netw. Open*, vol. 1, no. 5, p. e182327, Sep. 2018.

[53]   J. K. Kiecolt-Glaser, M. A. Belury, R. Andridge, W. B. Malarkey, and R. Glaser, "Omega-3 supplementation lowers inflammation and

anxiety in medical students: A randomized controlled trial," *Brain. Behav. Immun.*, vol. 25, no. 8, pp. 1725–1734, Nov. 2011.

[54] C. Williams and A. Garland, "Identifying and challenging unhelpful thinking," *Adv. Psychiatr. Treat.*, vol. 8, no. 5, pp. 377–386, Sep. 2002.

[55] S. M. Vanegas *et al.*, "Substituting whole grains for refined grains in a 6-wk randomized trial has a modest effect on gut microbiota and immune and inflammatory markers of healthy adults," *Am. J. Clin. Nutr.*, vol. 105, no. 3, pp. 635–650, Mar. 2017.

[56] A. Angioloni and C. Collar, "Nutritional and functional added value of oat, Kamut®, spelt, rye and buckwheat versus common wheat in breadmaking," *J. Sci. Food Agric.*, vol. 91, no. 7, pp. 1283–1292, May 2011.

[57] H. M. Roager *et al.*, "Whole grain-rich diet reduces body weight and systemic low-grade inflammation without inducing major changes of the gut microbiome: a randomised cross-over trial," *Gut*, vol. 68, no. 1, pp. 83–93, Jan. 2019.

[58] T. P. J. Solomon, F. F. Eves, and M. J. Laye, "Targeting Postprandial Hyperglycemia With Physical Activity May Reduce Cardiovascular Disease Risk. But What Should We Do, and When Is the Right Time to Move?," *Front. Cardiovasc. Med.*, vol. 5, p. 99, Jul. 2018.

[59] M. G. Flynn, M. M. Markofski, and A. E. Carrillo, "Elevated Inflammatory Status and Increased Risk of Chronic Disease in Chronological Aging: Inflamm-aging or Inflamm-inactivity?," *Aging Dis.*, vol. 10, no. 1, pp. 147–156, Feb. 2019.

[60] L. L. Toussaint, D. R. Williams, M. A. Musick, and S. A. Everson-Rose, "Why forgiveness may protect against depression: Hopelessness as an explanatory mechanism," *Personal. Ment. Health*, vol. 2, no. 2, pp. 89–103, Apr. 2008.

[61] N. J. Roese *et al.*, "Repetitive Regret, Depression,

and Anxiety: Findings from a Nationally Representative Survey," *J. Soc. Clin. Psychol.*, vol. 28, no. 6, pp. 671–688, Jun. 2009.

[62]   W. S. Tse and T. H. J. Yip, "Relationship among dispositional forgiveness of others, interpersonal adjustment and psychological well-being: Implication for interpersonal theory of depression," *Pers. Individ. Dif.*, vol. 46, no. 3, pp. 365–368, Feb. 2009.

[63]   W. Bruine de Bruin, A. Y. Dombrovski, A. M. Parker, and K. Szanto, "Late-life Depression, Suicidal Ideation, and Attempted Suicide: The Role of Individual Differences in Maximizing, Regret, and Negative Decision Outcomes," *J. Behav. Decis. Mak.*, vol. 29, no. 4, pp. 363–371, Oct. 2016.

[64]   G. L. Reed and R. D. Enright, "The effects of forgiveness therapy on depression, anxiety, and posttraumatic stress for women after spousal emotional abuse.," *J. Consult. Clin. Psychol.*, vol. 74, no. 5, pp. 920–9, Oct. 2006.

[65]   R. D. Enright and J. North, *Exploring forgiveness*. University of Wisconsin Press, 1998.

[66]   M. R. Monroe, J. J. Skowronski, W. Macdonald, and S. E. Wood, "The Mildly Depressed Experience More Post–Decisional Regret Than the Non–Depressed," *J. Soc. Clin. Psychol.*, vol. 24, no. 5, pp. 665–690, Aug. 2005.

[67]   J. K. Hirsch, J. R. Webb, and E. L. Jeglic, "Forgiveness, depression, and suicidal behavior among a diverse sample of college students," *J. Clin. Psychol.*, vol. 67, no. 9, pp. 896–906, Sep. 2011.